NAVIGATING CHANGES IN HEALTHCARE

*Managing Change Effectively for
Healthcare Professionals*

GIRISH BOMMAKANTI

STARDOM BOOKS

www.StardomBooks.com

STARDOM BOOKS
112 Bordeaux Ct.
Coppell, TX 75019, USA

FIRST EDITION AUGUST 2025

STARDOM BOOKS, LLC.
112 Bordeaux Ct. Coppell, TX 75019, USA

www.stardombooks.com

Stardom Books, United States
Stardom Alliance, India

NAVIGATING CHANGES IN HEALTHCARE
Managing Change Effectively for Healthcare Professionals

Girish Bommakanti

p. 338
cm. 13.5 X 21.5

Category: MED035000 : Medical : Health Care Delivery
MED011000: Medical : Caregiving
HEA028000: Health & Fitness : Health Care Issues

ISBN: 978-1-957456-75-1

DEDICATION

This book is dedicated to:
I owe my heartfelt gratitude to my brothers, Sudhir and
Samarendra Nath, whose encouragement has fueled my desire to
share my experiences and the work I've accomplished over the
last twenty-five years.
I am especially thankful to my mentor and reporting head,
Dr. N. Krishna Reddy, for his constant support and guidance
throughout these two decades.
My most profound appreciation goes to my wife, Silpa, for her
unwavering support and limitless encouragement.
My wonderful children, Hassi and Aanya, bring immense joy
and purpose to my life!
Fluffy, my faithful dog, has been an ever-present source of
comfort and joy during my long walks.
I am grateful to all my family members for their sustained
encouragement and relentless motivation.
Most importantly, I would like to thank my parents, whose
unwavering support and strength have been the
foundation of my journey.

ACKNOWLEDGMENTS

This book results from the unwavering support and contributions of many individuals who have enriched my journey. I am deeply grateful to each of them.

First and foremost, I extend my heartfelt thanks to my mentor, Dr. N. Krishna Reddy, whose guidance, wisdom, and encouragement over the past two decades have been invaluable. His insights have profoundly shaped both my work and this book.

I am equally grateful to my guide and professor, Dr. Alka Parikh, for her positive mentorship as a student and professionally. Her ability to transform daunting challenges into manageable opportunities has been genuinely inspiring.

To my brothers, Sudhir and Samarendra Nath, thank you for igniting my passion to share my story and your steadfast belief in my endeavors. Your encouragement has been a constant source of strength.

My deepest gratitude goes to my wife, Silpa, and my children, Hassi and Aanya, for their boundless love, patience, and support. You have been my anchor through the countless hours of writing and reflection.

I am immensely thankful to my parents, whose lifelong encouragement and sacrifices have made this achievement possible. Your strength and values continue to guide me.

Special thanks to the collaborators who generously shared their time and insights, enriching this book with valuable lessons: **Dr. N. Krishna Reddy, Dr. Alka Parikh, Dr. Ajay Bakshi, Col. M. Raj Gopal, Dr. Hala Zaid, Ratan Jalan, Farhad Ali, Dr. Shweta Singh, Dr. Priyesh Tiwari, Dr. Swapnil Kharnare, Dr. Dhaval Bhatt, and Bhavisha**. Your contributions have been instrumental.

To my colleagues and collaborators over the past two and a half decades and especially Access Health International team, thank you all for your insights, feedback, and camaraderie. Your contributions have enriched this work in countless ways.

I also thank the editorial and publishing team for their professionalism and dedication in bringing this book to life. Your expertise has been pivotal in shaping its final form.

My extended family and friends, thank you for your continuous support and motivation. Your belief in me has made this journey deeply meaningful.

I apologize for inadvertently omitting anyone who has contributed to this endeavor.

This book is a testament to the collective support of all those named and countless others who have touched my life.

Thank you.

CONTENTS

FOREWORD

Humans sought help to relieve their suffering from time immemorial. Healers emerged to meet this fundamental need of people. The art of healing has been evolving over the ages. A simple doctor-patient interaction has evolved into a highly complex health system with multiple actors and tools.

Even the basic hospital has evolved into a complex organization. In addition, health systems themselves are interconnected and interdependent with other social and environmental systems. The profession of health systems management has been constantly evolving in tandem with the development of health systems.

The doctor who establishes their clinic, nursing home, or small hospital starts managing their facilities. The public health professional cadre emerged to manage population health, unlike doctors, who focus on individual health as healthcare services expanded to include consultations involving generalists and specialists, as well as tests and treatments involving drugs and procedures, professionals specialized in management sciences were needed. Healthcare is a unique service, unlike others.

The core purpose of medicine has been to do no harm, relieve suffering, and prolong a healthy life. The core purpose of health systems is to respond to people's health and care needs when, where, and how they want, without causing financial hardships in accessing these services. Achieving these objectives efficiently, effectively, equitably, financially, and environmentally sustainably is one of the most significant challenges of managing healthcare services.

Balancing business and medical ethics has become challenging for people who lead and manage private for-profit healthcare enterprises.

Given the above context, the book by Girish Bommakanti is highly informative and timely. In this book, he attempts to distill insights from his rich experience, as well as insights from others who have succeeded in their unique ways, and insights from the scientific literature.

He tried to explore the qualities of leadership and techniques of change management. Blending of scientific outlook and practitioners' wisdom is the essence of this book. I am confident that both health management students and practicing professionals will find the book both unique and practical.

— Dr. N Krishna Reddy
CEO, Access Health International

PREFACE

My diverse experiences have shaped my deep-rooted commitment to healthcare transformation over the past 24 years. Having had the privilege of working with healthcare organizations across multiple countries, spanning both the private and public sectors, I have witnessed firsthand the intricate challenges institutions face—challenges that go beyond financial sustainability and operational constraints. These experiences have refined my perspective, strengthening my conviction that meaningful transformation in healthcare is not simply about policies and procedures; it is about leadership, culture, and the ability to implement sustainable change that lasts beyond immediate interventions.

Much of my career has been dedicated to working with healthcare organizations in crisis, particularly those struggling with financial sustainability. While financial distress often appeared to be the primary issue, deeper analysis revealed that money was merely a symptom of more profound structural inefficiencies, leadership gaps, and disengaged workforces. Institutions struggling with severe resource drain weren't just making poor financial decisions; they were often grappling with fragmented management processes, a lack of strategic direction, and an organizational culture resistant to change. Addressing these foundational challenges became the cornerstone of my work, allowing me to design turnaround strategies that not only stabilized organizations in the short term but also positioned them for long-term success.

In some cases, the solutions were straightforward, involving the identification of inefficiencies, optimization of resource allocation, or the implementation of strategic cost-cutting measures without compromising patient care. But more often than not, true transformation requires a shift in leadership mindset, rebuilding trust between management and frontline staff, and fostering a culture of accountability and innovation.

It wasn't just about fixing financial problems; it was about aligning people, processes, and purpose to create a healthcare environment that could evolve and sustain itself in an ever-changing landscape.

Beyond financial restructuring, my work in public health introduced me to the complexities of large-scale systemic change. Public health initiatives, despite being well-intentioned and supported by strategic frameworks, often struggle to bridge the gap between policy and execution. I have seen ambitious healthcare programs launched with enthusiasm, only to stall midway due to leadership transitions, bureaucratic inertia, or resistance from key stakeholders. New initiatives that looked promising on paper frequently unraveled when they encountered real-world healthcare environments, where workforce engagement was overlooked, and implementation lacked the necessary cultural integration.

These recurring patterns led me to a defining realization: the missing link in most healthcare transformation efforts is not the absence of good ideas but the failure to execute them effectively. Change management is often treated as an afterthought, yet it is the foundation upon which sustainable transformation must be built. A well-crafted strategic plan is meaningless if the people responsible for its execution are not engaged, equipped, and aligned with its objectives. Leadership is not just about making decisions at the top—it is about mobilizing an entire organization toward a shared vision, ensuring that every layer of the institution, from executives to frontline staff, is invested in long-term success.

Healthcare organizations worldwide are navigating an era of unprecedented complexity. The challenge of delivering high-quality care while maintaining financial viability has never been more daunting. Across hospitals, clinics, and public health institutions, leaders are grappling with the rapid pace of technological advancements, evolving patient expectations, and a constantly shifting regulatory landscape. In this volatile environment, two critical elements stand out as essential for an organization's ability to adapt and excel: effective leadership and the untapped potential of its workforce.

Strong leadership is the cornerstone of any healthcare transformation. However, leadership alone is not enough. It must be accompanied by the ability to manage change effectively, guiding institutions through transitions with precision, ensuring that new initiatives are seamlessly integrated into existing systems, and creating an environment where people embrace change rather than resist it. Managing transformation is not just about achieving short-term results; it is about embedding a culture of continuous improvement that ensures long-term sustainability. The process of leading change is as necessary as the change itself, and institutions that fail to recognize this reality often find themselves caught in cycles of stagnation and inefficiency.

Equally crucial is the role of the workforce in shaping the future of healthcare organizations. Despite being the backbone of the healthcare system, many professionals—whether doctors, nurses, administrators, public health managers, or support staff—are underutilized in organizational decision-making and change efforts. A hospital's most valuable resource is not its infrastructure or technology but the people who bring it to life every day. Yet, in many institutions, workforce engagement is an afterthought rather than a strategic priority. Unlocking the full potential of healthcare professionals requires more than just training and incentives—it demands leadership that empowers individuals at every level, fosters a culture of trust and accountability, and ensures that change management is not dictated from the top down but co-created with those on the frontlines. The road ahead for healthcare institutions is undeniably complex, but it is also rich with opportunity.

Those who embrace transformation, not as a reactionary measure but as a continuous journey, will be the ones who define the future of global health.

In the healthcare sector, organizations are not merely managing routine operations—they are navigating an ongoing evolution driven by technological breakthroughs, emerging diseases, shifting population health trends, and advancements in treatment modalities. The pace of change is relentless, demanding more than just reactive measures or short-term adjustments. While quick fixes and isolated interventions may provide temporary relief, they fail to create the resilience needed to sustain meaningful progress. To thrive in this ever-changing landscape, healthcare organizations must implement changes that are not only effective in the moment but also deeply embedded, holistically integrated, and institutionalized for long-term impact.

This is where sustainable change management becomes critical. Many change initiatives fail not because the ideas behind them are flawed but because they lack an integrated approach that aligns people, processes, culture, and systems. Transformation cannot be treated as a one-time project or a set of isolated improvements—it must be woven into the very fabric of an organization's operations and mindset. Every level of the organization, from senior leadership to frontline staff, must be engaged, equipped, and empowered to drive and sustain change. Without this alignment, even the most well-intentioned transformation efforts risk stagnation, inconsistency, or outright failure.

Sustainable change management extends far beyond financial sustainability; it is about addressing the core elements that define an organization's ability to evolve—its people, its culture, and its systems. Healthcare institutions that focus solely on short-term solutions or neglect the deeper cultural and systemic challenges may see initial success, but these gains will be temporary. True transformation requires a shift in how organizations think about change, moving beyond fragmented efforts and adopting a comprehensive approach that considers every element of the healthcare ecosystem—leadership, staff engagement, technology, and operational processes. Only by embracing this holistic perspective can healthcare organizations become truly adaptive and resilient.

The core question I seek to answer in this book is: How can healthcare professionals at all levels develop their leadership competencies and apply change management principles to create lasting, meaningful impact within their organizations?

The healthcare landscape is shifting faster than ever before. Those who can effectively manage and lead change will not only shape the future of their institutions but will also contribute to the broader evolution of global healthcare. This book is not just about theory—it provides practical, actionable tools to help you implement these concepts in your work environment, regardless of your role or level of experience.

If you apply the principles outlined in this book, I hope that you will undergo the following transformation:

You will gain a deeper understanding of change management concepts and their direct application to the healthcare industry.

You will develop the ability to lead change initiatives effectively, whether you are an aspiring leader or an experienced executive.

Your organization will benefit from sustainable transformation, yielding tangible results such as improved patient care, enhanced staff engagement, and greater financial stability.

Beyond individual leadership growth, this book contributes to a broader conversation about the future of healthcare. With the rapid acceleration of change—whether due to global health crises, technological innovation, or evolving patient expectations—the ability of healthcare organizations to adapt and innovate is more critical than ever. Leaders who can successfully guide transformation will be at the forefront of shaping a more sustainable, effective, and patient-centered healthcare system.

Each chapter of this book explores a distinct aspect of leadership and change management within healthcare organizations. By the time you reach the final page, you will have gained a comprehensive understanding of how to:

Recognize why leadership and change management are essential in today's healthcare landscape.

Apply change management frameworks effectively to your specific context, ensuring real-world impact.

The journey toward healthcare transformation is complex, but with the right tools, strategies, and leadership mindset, it is entirely achievable. This book is your guide to making that transformation a reality.

Strengthen your leadership competencies at every stage of your career, whether you are just beginning your journey or are a seasoned professional refining your expertise. The ability to lead effectively is not confined to a specific title or position—it is a skill that evolves and is essential at every level of healthcare.

Implement sustainable change strategies that create a lasting impact—whether in your immediate work environment, your healthcare organization, or a broader public health initiative. Transformation is not about temporary fixes; it is about embedding meaningful, lasting improvements that enhance both patient care and organizational resilience.

This book is designed to be both conceptual and practical, offering insights for those new to leadership and change management while providing deeper strategies for experienced professionals seeking to refine their approach. While you can read it cover-to-cover, I encourage you to engage with each chapter at a pace that aligns with your current understanding and professional needs.

Use the case studies and real-world examples as tools to bridge theory with application. Whether you manage a hospital, lead a clinic, or spearhead a public health initiative, the frameworks and strategies outlined here can be adapted to fit your unique challenges.

Think of this book as a guidebook rather than a manual—its value lies in how you apply its lessons to your specific context.

Take your time with each chapter. Don't rush through the material—pause to reflect on how these principles connect with the realities of your healthcare setting. Sustainable transformation doesn't happen overnight; it requires thoughtful planning, deliberate action, and a commitment to long-term impact. The more you internalize these lessons, the better equipped you will be to implement meaningful change.

At its core, this book is a call to action for healthcare professionals at every level. As you reach the final pages, please reflect on how you can apply these principles in your organization. Start small—choose one initiative that aligns with your institution's goals and take action. Even a minor improvement can catalyze greater transformation. Change begins with a single step, and momentum builds from there.

Healthcare transformation is not the responsibility of a select few—it requires leadership at every level, from frontline workers to senior executives. Whether you are directly leading a change initiative or supporting others in the process, I hope this book inspires you to take the lead as a change leader. Your ability to navigate and implement change will not only shape your organization's success but also contribute to the broader evolution of global healthcare.

The future of healthcare depends on leaders like you—those who understand the urgency of change management and are willing to take action to drive sustainable transformation.

Thank you for joining me on this journey to reimagine and revitalize healthcare. Let's get started.

— Girish Bommakanti

1

UNDERSTANDING THE HEALTHCARE ECOSYSTEM

U nderstanding the intricate and multifaceted healthcare ecosystem is crucial for achieving meaningful and sustainable transformation in today's rapidly evolving healthcare environment. The healthcare ecosystem encompasses a dynamic interplay of diverse components, including the public and private sectors, healthcare providers, patients, payers, regulators, policymakers, teaching institutions, and many other stakeholders.

These elements do not operate in isolation; they interact in complex, interdependent, and often unpredictable ways, influenced by economic forces, technological advancements, policy changes, and societal needs.

The healthcare ecosystem is a network designed to promote health, prevent disease, and provide care. However, the paths to achieving these objectives are shaped by a web of relationships and forces.

For instance, public and private entities collaborate and sometimes compete, while policymakers and regulators establish frameworks to ensure equitable access and safety.

At the same time, healthcare providers and payers negotiate financial models to sustain operations.

Patients, the ultimate beneficiaries, also play an increasingly active role, demanding transparency, convenience, and personalized care.

The interaction among these components determines the quality, cost, accessibility, and outcomes of healthcare services.

THE IMPORTANCE OF UNDERSTANDING THE ECOSYSTEM

Transforming healthcare does not merely involve introducing new technologies or changing policies; it requires a comprehensive understanding of how the system's components interconnect and influence one another.

For example, a new digital health platform may improve diagnostic accuracy; however, its success depends on factors such as provider adoption, patient engagement, regulatory approval, and payer reimbursement policies. Similarly, improving access to care might require aligning public funding with private sector delivery mechanisms, addressing systemic inequities, and fostering community partnerships.

Therefore, healthcare professionals, leaders, and policymakers must approach transformation from a systems perspective. Recognizing the dependencies and feedback loops within the ecosystem is essential for designing impactful and sustainable interventions.

As we delve deeper into the nuances of the healthcare ecosystem, it is essential to remember that transformation is both a science and an art. It requires evidence-based decision-making, strategic foresight, and empathy for those directly impacted by the system's performance. Understanding the healthcare ecosystem is not just an academic exercise but the first step in creating a more efficient, equitable, and patient-centered system.

THE STRUCTURE OF THE HEALTHCARE ECOSYSTEM

The healthcare ecosystem is a vast and intricate system that is broadly divided into two primary sectors: the public sector and the private sector. Each of these sectors plays a distinct yet interconnected role in delivering healthcare services, shaping policies, and ensuring the overall functioning of the system.

Understanding the structure of these sectors and their respective roles is essential for grasping the dynamics of the ecosystem.

The Public Sector

The public sector serves as the backbone of the healthcare system in many countries, focusing on ensuring equitable access to healthcare services for all citizens.

Characterized by government ownership, funding, and regulation, the public sector often operates large-scale healthcare infrastructure, including hospitals, community clinics, and public health initiatives. Its primary goal is to safeguard public health through preventive measures, disease control, and the provision of essential services.

Key features of the public sector include:

- **Universal Access**: Providing care that is accessible to all, regardless of income or social status.
- **Public Funding**: Healthcare services are typically financed through taxation or government-subsidized programs.
- **Regulation and Oversight**: Establishing policies, standards, and guidelines to ensure safety, quality, and equity.

For example, in the United Kingdom, the National Health Service (NHS) is a publicly funded system that provides comprehensive care to residents, free at the point of use.

It is a model of how the public sector can deliver universal healthcare while striking a balance between cost efficiency and broad accessibility.

CASE STUDY: THAILAND'S UNIVERSAL COVERAGE SCHEME (UCS)

Thailand achieved Universal Health Coverage (UHC) in 2002, with its entire population covered under one of three public health insurance schemes:

- **Civil Servant Medical Benefit Scheme (CSMBS)**: Primarily for government employees and their dependents.
- **Social Health Insurance (SHI)**: Employment-based coverage for private-sector workers.
- **Universal Coverage Scheme (UCS)**: A non-contributory scheme ensuring entitlement to health care for all Thai citizens.

The UCS has played a pivotal role in improving access to health care and providing financial risk protection, resulting in a significant reduction in catastrophic health spending and impoverishment among Thai households.

Structure and Financing of UCS

The UCS is managed by the National Health Security Office (NHSO) and funded through a publicly financed, non-contributory model. Key features include:

- **Comprehensive Benefits Package**: Covers outpatient care, inpatient care, high-cost treatments, preventive services, and health promotion.
- **Full Cost Subsidy**: The UCS budget accounts for labor, materials, and capital depreciation costs, eliminating the need for co-payments or balance billing.

To ensure sustainability, the UCS uses closed-end provider payment systems, such as:

- Age-Adjusted Capitation for outpatient care.
- Diagnosis-Related Groups (DRG) under a global budget for inpatient care.
- Direct Negotiations for high-cost medicines and medical devices, leveraging NHSO's monopsonistic purchasing power.

This budgeting approach prevents overspending, as UCS is expected to fully utilize its finite resources allocated for its 48.787 million members.

Outcomes and Achievements

- **Access to Health Care**: The UCS has provided universal entitlement, ensuring that even unemployed individuals or dependents of CSMBS members who lose coverage are automatically enrolled in UCS. It has particularly benefited vulnerable groups, including low-income populations and rural residents.
- **Financial Risk Protection**: Thailand has achieved a low prevalence of catastrophic health spending and impoverishment compared to other middle-income countries. Balance billing is strictly prohibited, ensuring that no unexpected financial burdens are placed on UCS members.
- **Efficiency and Cost Control:** The NHSO has implemented rigorous cost management through its monopsony, securing favorable prices for high-cost medicines and medical devices. Savings from negotiations have been reinvested to expand service coverage for UCS members.

Challenges and Policy Coherence

Despite the successes of UCS, Thailand faces challenges in harmonizing its three public health insurance schemes:

- **Inefficiencies in CSMBS**: The CSMBS operates on a fee-for-service model for outpatient care and utilizes 27 bands of DRG weights for inpatient care, lacking a global budget, which leads to disproportionately higher spending. Per capita expenditure for CSMBS is approximately four times higher than for UCS, raising concerns about equity and efficiency.

- **Policy Incoherence**: Differences in price setting, purchasing, and regulation between CSMBS, SHI, and UCS create inefficiencies.

Recommendations for Improvement

- **Enhancing Policy Integration**: Harmonize purchasing mechanisms and pricing strategies across CSMBS, SHI, and UCS to reduce disparities and inefficiencies.
- **Strengthening Governance**: Establish unified oversight to ensure equitable resource distribution and adherence to best practices across all schemes.
- **Expanding Cost-Effectiveness Strategies**: Continue leveraging monopsonistic purchasing power to negotiate better prices for high-cost interventions.
- Invest in preventive care and primary healthcare systems to reduce reliance on high-cost tertiary care.
- **Increasing Public Awareness and Engagement**: Empower citizens to understand their entitlements under UCS and other schemes, fostering accountability and trust in the health system.

Thailand's Universal Coverage Scheme demonstrates how a middle-income country can achieve significant milestones in health care access and financial protection. The UCS model, characterized by its comprehensive benefits package, efficient cost control measures, and strict financial protections, has set a global benchmark for UHC implementation. However, addressing inefficiencies and policy incoherence among the three public health schemes is crucial to sustaining Thailand's progress and ensuring equitable health outcomes for all citizens.

The Private Sector

The private sector complements the public sector by offering specialized, innovative, and often more flexible healthcare services. It consists of privately owned hospitals, clinics, pharmaceutical companies, insurance providers, and technology firms. While many private healthcare entities operate on a for-profit basis, the sector also includes non-profit organizations that focus on specific health needs.

Key features of the private sector include:

- **Market-Driven Innovation**: Investment in cutting-edge technologies, research, and personalized medicine.
- **Efficiency and Choice**: Providing patients with a range of options and shorter wait times compared to public systems.
- **Competitive Pricing**: While private healthcare can lead to higher costs, competition often drives improvements in service quality and efficiency.

Private sector contributions are evident globally. In the United States, organizations such as the Mayo Clinic and Kaiser Permanente illustrate how private institutions can combine innovation with high-quality care delivery. In India, the private sector plays a dominant role in healthcare delivery, with networks like Apollo Hospitals and Fortis Healthcare providing advanced medical treatments and reaching underserved populations through digital health platforms. Similarly, in Egypt, private healthcare providers have expanded significantly, with institutions like Alameda Hospital Group leading efforts in modernizing services, integrating technology, and increasing access in urban and semi-urban areas.

The Full Spectrum of Healthcare Stakeholders

Together with the public sector, the private healthcare industry plays a vital role in shaping health outcomes, but it is only one part of a much larger ecosystem.

Effective healthcare delivery relies on the coordinated efforts of various stakeholders, including government agencies, private healthcare providers, life sciences companies, universities, research and development organizations, Policymakers, and non-profit providers, as well as patients themselves Understanding the contributions of each is crucial to comprehending how the system operates and evolves.

Key Players in the Healthcare Ecosystem

- **Government Agencies**: Develop and enforce health policies, manage public health campaigns, and fund healthcare infrastructure.
- **Private Organizations**: Deliver healthcare services, develop new treatments, and manage insurance plans.
- **Non-Profit Organizations**: Advocate for health equity, conduct research, and support underserved populations.
- **Patients:** Patients play an increasingly active role as informed consumers, shaping demand and influencing the design of the healthcare system.

Interactions Between Sectors

The public and private sectors often interact in both collaborative and competitive ways. **Public-private partnerships (PPPs)** have become increasingly common, enabling governments and private organizations to collaborate on enhancing service delivery.

For example, governments may outsource diagnostic lab services to private providers or partner with private organizations to manage large-scale vaccination campaigns.

- **Real-World Example:** A strong illustration of public-private collaboration is India's **Ayushman Bharat Pradhan Mantri Jan Arogya Yojana** (PM-JAY), a government-funded health insurance scheme designed to provide free secondary and tertiary care to vulnerable populations.

- While the public sector manages the scheme, private hospitals are empaneled to deliver care, demonstrating how public funding and private sector efficiency can work together to expand access to healthcare.

By understanding the structure of the healthcare ecosystem—including the distinctive yet interdependent roles of the public and private sectors—healthcare professionals can better navigate the challenges and opportunities in delivering care. The interactions between these sectors, along with contributions from key stakeholders, highlight the complexity of the system and the need for thoughtful, strategic transformation efforts.

CHALLENGES AND OPPORTUNITIES IN THE HEALTHCARE ECOSYSTEM

The healthcare ecosystem operates within a dynamic and complex environment shaped by persistent challenges and emerging opportunities. While systemic issues such as funding shortages, inequities in access to care, and regulatory hurdles remain obstacles, advancements in technology, cross-sector collaboration, and innovative funding mechanisms offer significant avenues for transformation. Addressing these challenges while leveraging opportunities is essential to building a resilient, efficient, and equitable healthcare system.

Challenges in the Healthcare Ecosystem

One of the primary challenges in the healthcare sector is **inadequate and fragmented funding mechanisms**, which hinder the delivery of consistent and equitable care. This issue is particularly pronounced in low-income and rural areas, where underfunded public health programs struggle to meet community needs.

For example,

- **Sub-Saharan Africa**: Underfunding drives 50% of global maternal deaths and 25% of child deaths.
- **South Asia**: Afghanistan and Nepal face similar crises, with underfunded systems fueling polio and TB.
- **Fragile States**: Yemen and South Sudan need emergency funding and community-based care to stabilize systems.

Another significant challenge is **inequitable access to healthcare services**, often determined by socioeconomic status, geography, and systemic barriers. Research has shown that a person's zip code can be a stronger predictor of health outcomes than their genetic code. For instance, rural communities often lack access to specialized care, resulting in poorer health outcomes compared to urban populations. These disparities highlight the critical need for targeted interventions to bridge healthcare accessibility gaps.

Regulatory hurdles also complicate efforts to innovate and streamline care. **Overlapping jurisdictions, inconsistent policies, and bureaucratic delays** can slow the adoption of technologies such as telemedicine, which has the potential to expand access to care, particularly for underserved populations. Without streamlined regulatory frameworks, healthcare systems may struggle to integrate digital solutions efficiently, delaying critical advancements in patient care.

TECHNOLOGICAL INNOVATION

Digital transformation in healthcare extends far beyond artificial intelligence, encompassing a broad suite of technologies that are reshaping how care is delivered, accessed, and managed. Innovations such as telemedicine, mobile health applications, electronic health records (EHRs), remote monitoring devices, and digital therapeutics are enhancing patient engagement, expanding access to care, particularly in rural and underserved areas, and improving system efficiency.

These tools enable providers to deliver more personalized, timely, and coordinated care while empowering patients to actively participate in managing their health. As digital health ecosystems mature, they serve as the foundation upon which more advanced technologies, such as AI, can be effectively deployed and scaled.

Advances in artificial intelligence (AI), data analytics, and telehealth present transformative opportunities for improving healthcare delivery.

AI-powered diagnostics, for example, have demonstrated enhanced accuracy in early disease detection, particularly in conditions such as cancer, which can potentially save lives and reduce treatment costs. Similarly, predictive analytics, which leverages real-time and nontraditional data sources, enables public health agencies to anticipate disease outbreaks and allocate resources more effectively (Deloitte, 2024).

CROSS-SECTOR COLLABORATION

Public-private partnerships (PPPs) provide a promising avenue for overcoming systemic limitations by leveraging the strengths of both sectors. While the public sector provides scale and accessibility, the private sector drives efficiency and innovation. One of the most notable examples of PPPs in action was the global distribution of COVID-19 vaccines, where governments, pharmaceutical companies, and logistics firms worked together to ensure widespread and equitable access. This collaboration underscored the effectiveness of collaborative efforts in addressing global healthcare challenges.

- **Payer Systems Integrations**: The integration of payer systems' data in healthcare involves connecting and harmonizing data from various sources, such as electronic health records (EHRs), claims databases, provider networks, and patient-reported outcomes, to create a unified, actionable dataset for health insurers (also known as payors). This integration aims to enhance decision-making, improve patient outcomes, streamline operations, and support value-based care models.

- **Localization of Pharmaceuticals and Medical Devices in Countries:** The localization of pharmaceuticals and medical devices offers transformative opportunities to enhance healthcare access, ensure compliance, and drive economic benefits across countries. By addressing regulatory, cultural, and logistical challenges through strategic localization, companies can unlock new markets, improve patient outcomes, and contribute to resilient healthcare systems. For instance, aligning with Saudi Arabia's localization goals, Singapore's bio-cluster, etc

- **Workforce Capacity Building**: Workforce capacity building in healthcare presents a critical opportunity to address global shortages, enhance care quality, and support resilient health systems. By investing in training, upskilling, and retaining healthcare workers, countries can enhance patient outcomes, meet the growing demand, and reap economic benefits.

- **Healthcare Delivery Models – Reinvention**: Reinventing healthcare delivery models presents opportunities to enhance access, efficiency, and outcomes through digital, value-based, and decentralized approaches. These models intersect with payor systems integration (data sharing), pharmaceutical localization (culturally relevant care), and workforce capacity building (training for new systems). By addressing challenges such as interoperability and equity, stakeholders can transform the healthcare system.

REIMAGINING THE HEALTH ECOSYSTEM: PROGRAMS, POLICIES, AND SYSTEMS FOR STRENGTHENING PUBLIC HEALTH

The limitations of traditional public health systems have been starkly revealed in recent years, from pandemic response gaps to growing health inequities and the increasing burden of chronic diseases. As populations grow and challenges such as climate change, urbanization, and digital disruption accelerate, health systems can no longer afford to operate in silos. There is a pressing need to reimagine the intersection of healthcare, governance, and community well-being—and to build public health systems that are resilient, equitable, and future-ready.

A Vision for Public Health Transformation

For decades, public health leaders have envisioned a transformed system that shifts the focus from reactive care to proactive prevention. In this reimagined ecosystem, healthcare would prioritize predicting and preventing illness at the community level, thereby reducing healthcare costs and improving outcomes through systemic changes and cross-sector coordination. However, achieving this vision is far from simple. Socioeconomic factors—such as a person's zip code—often play a larger role in determining health outcomes than their genetic code (Deloitte Center for Health Solutions & Government Insights, 2024).

The present moment offers unique opportunities to reform public health systems, driven by heightened public attention and increased government funding. However, these opportunities are counterbalanced by significant challenges, including funding backlogs, chronic disease epidemics, climate change, and systemic inequities. Addressing these issues requires a strategic, multidimensional approach to reshape the public health landscape and build resilience within the system.

THE ROLE OF CONNECTED THINKING
IN HEALTHCARE

Healthcare systems are becoming increasingly interconnected with macroeconomic megatrends, geopolitical shifts, and technological advancements. BMI's "Connected Thinking" approach exemplifies this integration, combining expertise across multiple sectors with political and economic analysis. By incorporating insights from pharmaceuticals, medical devices, telecommunications, and IT, Connected Thinking offers a holistic perspective on healthcare dynamics (BMI, 2023).

This interdisciplinary approach highlights how external forces shape healthcare systems. For example, the transition to low-carbon energy affects healthcare supply chains, while geopolitical tensions influence global trade in medical technologies. Understanding these interdependencies underscores the importance of adaptable and resilient healthcare strategies.

External Forces Influencing Healthcare

- **Macroeconomic Megatrends**: Healthcare spending, particularly in developed markets, has been affected by slowing economic growth and tighter fiscal policies. However, emerging markets are driving growth in health expenditure, investing heavily in health system resilience and digital health technologies following the COVID-19 pandemic.
- **Technological Transformation**: The rapid digitalization of healthcare is reshaping service delivery, with telemedicine, artificial intelligence (AI), and genomic medicine at the forefront. AI's potential in diagnostics and drug discovery is revolutionizing precision medicine, improving patient outcomes despite challenges related to data quality and integration with legacy systems.

- **Geopolitical and Trade Tensions**: Global uncertainties, including the aftermath of the COVID-19 pandemic and Russia's invasion of Ukraine, have underscored the importance of resilient healthcare systems. These geopolitical shifts have also affected medical device and pharmaceutical supply chains, creating both risks and opportunities for healthcare stakeholders.
- **Low Carbon Transition**: The healthcare sector is increasingly recognizing its role in global sustainability efforts. Investments in energy-efficient infrastructure, eco-friendly practices, and carbon-neutral healthcare delivery models are aligning healthcare operations with climate action goals, ensuring sustainable yet high-quality care.
- **Investment Trends in Healthcare**: The non-cyclical nature of the healthcare market makes it highly attractive to investors. Financial institutions, pharmaceutical companies, consulting firms, and IT enterprises are investing in high-margin innovations, including surgical robots, AI-driven diagnostics, and wearable health monitoring devices. With aging populations and rising global healthcare demands, these investment trends are expected to accelerate further.

Healthcare Expenditure and GDP

Healthcare expenditure reflects the scale and priorities of a nation's healthcare system. Countries where healthcare spending constitutes a high percentage of GDP often present fertile ground for growth in pharmaceuticals, medical devices, and digital health innovations. These nations typically benefit from robust infrastructure, favorable regulatory environments, and strong collaboration between governments, academic institutions, and private companies.

For example, Sweden and Canada, recognized leaders in digital health, benefit from high healthcare investment as a percentage of GDP, which fosters innovation in telemedicine, electronic health records (EHRs), and data-driven healthcare solutions (BMI, 2023). Prioritizing healthcare spending allows these countries to attract investment, develop a skilled workforce, and establish a supportive environment for research and development (R&D).

Healthcare systems in nations with high health expenditure relative to GDP present unique opportunities for pharmaceutical and medical device companies. Key benefits include:

- **Favorable Regulations**: Streamlined approval processes for introducing innovative medical products and technologies.
- **Research Collaboration**: Increased investment in R&D partnerships between academia, private enterprises, and government agencies.
- **Skilled Workforce**: Access to a strong pool of trained healthcare professionals, fostering high-quality patient care and medical innovation.

For example, the United States spends over 17% of its GDP on healthcare, creating an environment that supports medical breakthroughs, advanced care delivery models, and cutting-edge pharmaceutical innovations.

Government-Funded Healthcare

Government-funded healthcare systems emphasize universal access, cost control, and efficiency. By negotiating prices and centralizing administrative functions, these systems achieve economies of scale, redirecting savings toward patient care and public health initiatives.

A key example is the UK's National Health Service (NHS), which provides universal access to healthcare despite challenges such as funding constraints and wait times for non-urgent care (BMI, 2023).

Similarly, Sweden's government-funded healthcare model ensures comprehensive coverage for all citizens, with a focus on preventive care and efforts to minimize health disparities.

However, government-funded systems require balancing trade-offs, such as higher taxes or potential inefficiencies in resource allocation. Countries with government-dominated healthcare systems must continually adapt their policies and funding mechanisms to maintain equity, accessibility, and operational efficiency.

Emerging Market Dynamics

Healthcare expenditure growth in emerging markets remains strong, driven by post-COVID-19 investments and efforts to enhance the resilience of healthcare systems. Many emerging economies are prioritizing digitalization and expanding access to universal healthcare, particularly in the Asia-Pacific and Latin America regions.

Investments in health infrastructure, such as new hospitals, clinics, and telehealth solutions, aim to close access gaps and improve care quality (BMI, 2023). These markets also present substantial opportunities for pharmaceutical and medical device companies, driven by increasing demand for innovative treatments and advanced medical technologies.

However, significant disparities in healthcare access and funding persist between urban and rural areas, posing challenges to the equitable distribution of healthcare. Addressing these disparities requires targeted policy interventions, private-sector engagement, and infrastructure expansion to ensure sustainable healthcare improvements.

The Continuum of Care

The continuum of care aims to optimize patient outcomes by ensuring seamless transitions across healthcare providers and settings. This approach emphasizes the delivery of timely, appropriate care, reducing complications, and enhancing quality of life.

Medical device firms and pharmaceutical companies play a pivotal role in supporting this continuum by developing tools for monitoring and managing patient health across various stages of care. For example, innovations in remote monitoring and targeted therapies enable more personalized and effective care, particularly for chronic diseases. By addressing patient needs holistically, the continuum of care fosters better health outcomes while simultaneously reducing healthcare costs.

The continuum of care concept emphasizes coordinated healthcare delivery across various providers and settings to improve patient outcomes:

- **Medical Devices**: Innovations like remote monitoring tools enable ongoing care for chronic conditions.
- **Pharmaceuticals**: Drugs tailored to prevention, treatment, and recovery phases enhance the patient journey.

Example: Diabetic patients benefit from integrated care models that include wearable glucose monitors, insulin delivery devices, and patient education programs, ensuring continuous monitoring and proactive management.

Macroeconomic Themes in Healthcare: The healthcare sector's response to macroeconomic challenges, such as slowing growth and fiscal tightening, is multifaceted:

- **Digital Health Investment**: Nations with robust digital strategies, such as Sweden and Canada, lead the way in integrating telemedicine and electronic health records (EHRs) into their healthcare systems.
- **Focus on Mental and Elderly Care**: Fiscal constraints are balanced by targeted support for mental health services and aging populations.

- **Digital Health Technologies:** Digital health is among the fastest-growing subsectors, driven by advancements in AI, telemedicine, and health apps.
AI-accelerated drug discovery offers high-return potential, though challenges such as regulatory compliance and data quality remain significant barriers.
Example: Sweden's digital health market illustrates the impact of cohesive national strategies in driving adoption and fostering innovation.
- **Health Infrastructure:** The demand for modernized hospitals and clinics is increasing, particularly in the Asia-Pacific region and other emerging markets. Developed markets benefit from advanced healthcare technologies, such as robotic surgery and virtual reality-based medical training, while low-income nations continue to struggle with resource disparities.

Challenges:
- Outdated healthcare facilities and unequal regional access to quality care.
- Rising healthcare costs are associated with chronic diseases and aging populations.

Opportunities: Adoption of electronic health records (EHRs) and telemedicine solutions to streamline operations and improve access to care.

The healthcare ecosystem is undergoing profound changes, driven by external forces, technological advancements, and shifting macroeconomic realities. Strategies like BMI's Connected Thinking approach are essential for navigating these complexities and identifying opportunities in a rapidly evolving market. Bridging disparities, embracing innovation, and fostering cross-sector collaboration will be critical in achieving a more equitable and resilient healthcare future.

The Future of Global Health and Healthcare: Shaping a Resilient, Equitable, and Sustainable System

In recent years, the global healthcare system has faced unprecedented disruptions, including the COVID-19 pandemic and ongoing challenges in geopolitics, economics, and the environment.

These crises have hindered progress toward health-related Sustainable Development Goals (SDGs), exacerbated inequalities, and increased pressure on already overburdened healthcare systems.

Despite these setbacks, the World Economic Forum, in collaboration with L.E.K. Consulting, has developed a strategic outlook for the future of global health and healthcare. This vision emphasizes equity, resilience, innovation, and sustainability as the core pillars essential for transforming global healthcare systems.

The following sections outline these pillars and the barriers that must be overcome to achieve meaningful change.

Equitable Access and Outcomes

A future-focused vision for healthcare must prioritize equitable access to healthcare services and improved health outcomes for all. This pillar emphasizes the importance of fair distribution of key health determinants, including:

- Nutrition
- Education
- Sanitation
- Healthcare services

Ensuring equitable access means that all individuals, particularly vulnerable populations, can receive the care they need to lead healthy lives. However, achieving equity in health outcomes requires addressing systemic inequalities that disproportionately affect:

- Lower-income communities
- Racial and ethnic minorities

- Underserved populations in remote or rural areas

One of the significant challenges in achieving equitable healthcare access lies in the underrepresentation of specific populations in health data. Without accurate and comprehensive data that reflects population diversity, it becomes difficult to identify and address disparities in care delivery and health outcomes. To bridge this gap, policymakers and healthcare leaders must implement strategies that:

- Ensure all communities are adequately represented in health data collection and research.
- Develop inclusive policies that provide equal access to healthcare regardless of socioeconomic background.
- Offer affordable and culturally competent care, closing gaps in health equity and ensuring that all individuals receive high-quality treatment tailored to their needs.

As health systems evolve, it is crucial to ensure that everyone, especially vulnerable groups, has access to the fundamental determinants of health.

Universal Health Coverage (UHC) plays a pivotal role in this process, reinforcing the principle that health services should be available to all people, regardless of their ability to pay.

CASE STUDY: TRACKING UNIVERSAL HEALTH COVERAGE (UHC) PROGRESS IN 2023

Universal Health Coverage (UHC) is a cornerstone of the United Nations' Sustainable Development Goal (SDG) 3.8, aimed at ensuring access to essential health services and financial protection for all by 2030. However, the latest report by the World Health Organization (WHO) and the World Bank Group highlights stagnation in progress towards UHC globally, emphasizing both challenges and opportunities for accelerating advancements.

Current Status and Challenges

1. Service Coverage Stagnation:

- Since 2015, global progress in UHC service coverage has slowed significantly. The UHC Service Coverage Index (SCI) increased marginally from 65 in 2015 to 68 in 2021.
- Approximately 4.5 billion people worldwide lacked access to essential health services in 2021, with low-income countries (LICs) and lower-middle-income countries (LMICs) experiencing the most significant gaps in access.

2. Financial Hardship:

- The incidence of catastrophic out-of-pocket (OOP) health spending, which exceeds 10% of household budgets, has increased.
- In 2019, 1.3 billion people faced impoverishing health spending at relative poverty lines, and 344 million at extreme poverty lines.

3. Persistent Inequalities:

- Service coverage disparities exist within and between countries. Vulnerable populations, particularly rural and impoverished households, remain disproportionately excluded from essential health services.
- Financial protection is undermined by heavy reliance on OOP health spending, especially in LICs and LMICs.

4. Impact of COVID-19:

- The pandemic exacerbated financial hardships and disrupted global health service delivery.
- Between 2019 and 2021, UHC progress stalled due to the diversion of resources to COVID-19-related services.

Key Insights and Opportunities

1. Service Coverage Trends:

- Infectious disease treatment, such as HIV and

tuberculosis care, has shown significant progress. However, non-communicable diseases (NCDs) and reproductive, maternal, newborn, and child health (RMNCH) require greater investment to achieve UHC targets.

- Strengthening primary health care (PHC) systems is crucial for expanding access to essential services and reducing disparities.

2. Financial Protection Imperatives:

- High OOP health spending remains a significant barrier to financial protection. Innovative financing mechanisms, such as pre-paid pooled funds and reduced user charges, are critical.
- Exempting low-income and vulnerable populations from OOP payments can mitigate poverty and financial hardship.

3. Policy and Governance:

- Achieving UHC requires a political commitment and deliberate policy action, including the reallocation of resources to the health sector and an increase in public health funding.
- Countries must prioritize investments in primary health care (PHC) and expand the scope of primary care services to include diagnostic and treatment options.

4. The Role of Partnerships:

- Collaboration with multilateral agencies, civil society, and the private sector is essential for building resilient health systems.
- Targeted efforts should leverage global initiatives, such as the WHO UHC Billion target, to improve service coverage and financial protection simultaneously.

Recommendations
1. Accelerate Service Expansion:

- Focus on underperforming areas such as NCDs and

RMNCH to ensure holistic improvements in service coverage.

- Invest in Primary Health Care (PHC) to strengthen health systems and bridge gaps in rural and underserved communities.

2. Enhance Financial Protection:

- Limit OOP spending through fixed, low, or capped co-payments for essential services and medicines.
- Develop social safety nets and contingency funds to protect households from financial shocks during health crises.

3. Strengthen Governance:

- Incorporate UHC into national health strategies and ensure sustained political leadership to achieve the SDG 3.8 goals.
- Utilize robust data and evidence to monitor progress and adjust strategies as necessary.

4. Leverage Post-COVID Recovery:

- Build on the lessons learned from COVID-19 to enhance health system resilience, prioritizing resources for pandemic preparedness and public health emergencies.
- Protect public health budgets from economic downturns by exploring diversified and innovative funding models that support sustainable growth.

The 2023 UHC Monitoring Report underscores the urgent need for accelerated action to meet the 2030 UHC targets. While substantial progress has been made in infectious disease control, broader and more equitable advancements in service coverage and financial protection are critical. Achieving Universal Health Coverage (UHC) is ultimately a political and economic choice, requiring effective leadership, robust financing, and inclusive health policies. The time to act is now to ensure health for all, leaving no one behind.

HEALTHCARE SYSTEM TRANSFORMATION

The second pillar focuses on transforming healthcare systems to become more resilient and capable of providing high-quality care in both expected and unexpected circumstances.

The COVID-19 pandemic exposed the fragility of healthcare systems worldwide, underscoring the urgent need for structural resilience within health systems.

Resilience involves ensuring that healthcare systems can:

- Manage future pandemics and emergencies effectively.
- Sustain regular operations and adapt to evolving population needs.
- A transformed healthcare system must prioritize:
- The integration of new technologies to enhance efficiency and patient care.
- A well-supported workforce capable of delivering high-quality care.
- Infrastructure improvements to strengthen healthcare accessibility and operational efficiency.

Many healthcare systems today suffer from fragmented services, leading to inefficiencies and poor patient outcomes. By adopting integrated care models, healthcare providers can:

- Improve coordination among different care providers.
- Enhance continuity of care for better patient experiences.
- Shift towards patient-centered care, empowering individuals to take an active role in their health decisions.

Addressing Workforce Challenges

A key aspect of healthcare system transformation is tackling workforce shortages and burnout.

In recent years, healthcare professionals have faced unprecedented stress and overwhelming workloads, resulting in:

- High rates of burnout and mental health challenges.
- Increased staff turnover, leading to workforce shortages.
- Reduced quality of care due to fatigue and emotional exhaustion.

To ensure the future resilience of healthcare systems, it is crucial to:

- Improve working conditions and invest in staff well-being.
- Expand training opportunities to develop a skilled workforce.
- Foster a culture of support and mental health awareness within the healthcare sector.

Technology and Innovation

Technology and innovation are key drivers of healthcare transformation, particularly in:

- Enhancing patient care through data-driven decision-making.
- Increasing accessibility to medical services via digital health tools.
- Reducing healthcare costs by improving efficiency and resource allocation.

The integration of digital health tools, artificial intelligence (AI), and big data analytics is enabling healthcare providers to deliver:

- More precise and personalized treatments.Improved diagnostic accuracy through AI-assisted imaging and analysis.
- Optimized resource management to prevent inefficiencies.
- As the healthcare sector accelerates its digital transformation, it is essential to:

- Develop funding models that support the implementation and scaling of innovative solutions.
- Ensure telemedicine adoption continues to extend care access to remote and underserved populations.
- Leverage AI and machine learning to predict patient outcomes and enhance personalized treatment plans.

Managing the Challenges of Technological Adoption

While technology presents tremendous opportunities, its adoption must be carefully managed to prevent unintended consequences.

Key challenges include:

- Data privacy and security concerns require robust cybersecurity measures.
- Interoperability issues, ensuring seamless integration between new and existing systems.
- Digital literacy barriers, as healthcare providers and patients must be trained to use new technologies effectively.

To maximize the benefits of healthcare innovation, policies must be in place to:

- Protect patient data while ensuring the ethical use of AI.
- Facilitate interoperability to ensure the seamless integration of digital health solutions.
- Promote digital education and training among healthcare professionals and patients to enhance their understanding and improve patient care.

ENVIRONMENTAL SUSTAINABILITY IN HEALTHCARE

The environmental sustainability pillar addresses the healthcare sector's impact on climate change and its role in promoting public health through environmental responsibility. Healthcare systems worldwide contribute significantly to:

- Medical waste production includes hazardous and non-hazardous waste.
- Carbon emissions from hospital operations, energy use, and medical supply chains.
- High energy consumption, particularly in extensive medical facilities and equipment usage.

The Urgency of Sustainable Healthcare Practices

- Mitigating climate change and its effects on global health.
- Improving overall public health outcomes, as air pollution, water contamination, and environmental hazards directly impact population health.
- Reducing long-term healthcare costs is crucial, as preventable diseases linked to poor environmental conditions increase the burden on healthcare systems.

Key Strategies for Sustainable Healthcare

- Implementing energy-efficient infrastructure in hospitals and clinics.
- Reducing medical waste through improved waste management and eco-friendly alternatives.
- Encouraging the use of sustainable medical supplies and promoting environmentally responsible pharmaceutical practices.
- Promoting climate-resilient health policies that protect vulnerable populations from environmental health risks.

As healthcare organizations strive to align their operations with global sustainability goals, integrating green initiatives will become an essential part of a future-proofed, resilient healthcare system.

Hospitals, clinics, and other healthcare facilities should adopt sustainable practices, including:

- Reducing energy consumption through efficient hospital infrastructure and renewable energy sources.
- Increasing recycling efforts and implementing better waste management systems.
- Minimizing the environmental impact of pharmaceuticals and medical supplies by adopting sustainable procurement and disposal practices.

Moreover, the healthcare sector must proactively prepare for and address the health impacts of climate change, such as:

- The rise in vector-borne diseases is due to shifting climate conditions.
- Heat-related illnesses disproportionately affect vulnerable populations.
- The increased frequency of natural disasters necessitates a resilient healthcare infrastructure and effective emergency response strategies.

ADDRESSING BARRIERS TO TRANSFORMATION

Case studies from around the world highlight several key challenges that hinder healthcare transformation:

1. Global Health Disparities: The widening gap in healthcare access between developed and developing nations remains a significant barrier to achieving equitable health outcomes. To bridge this gap, innovations must be inclusive and adaptable to different economic and cultural contexts.

2. Regulatory Challenges: The slow pace of regulatory change often limits the speed at which new healthcare innovations can be deployed. Regulatory frameworks must evolve to:

- Accommodate emerging technologies, such as AI-driven diagnostics and digital therapeutics.
- Support new business models that enhance healthcare accessibility and affordability.

3. Lack of Collaboration: Fragmented efforts between key stakeholders—governments, private sector players, and civil society organizations—often slow progress. Stronger collaboration is essential to scaling healthcare solutions, including:

- Public-private partnerships (PPPs) to drive investment and innovation.
- Cross-industry collaboration, integrating expertise from tech, pharma, and finance.
- Global cooperation, ensuring healthcare innovations reach underserved regions.

4. Workforce Shortages: The healthcare workforce crisis is a growing concern. Sustainable solutions are needed to:

- Improve training programs and career pathways to attract new talent.
- Enhance retention strategies by offering better compensation, mental health support, and professional development opportunities.
- Address workforce burnout by creating supportive and resilient work environments.

5. The Digital Divide: As digital health innovations continue to expand, it is crucial to ensure that they reach all populations, particularly in low-income regions. Barriers such as limited digital literacy and inadequate infrastructure must be addressed through:

- Investments in broadband connectivity and mobile health platforms.
- Digital education initiatives to empower both patients and healthcare professionals.

The Path Forward: Building a Resilient, Sustainable, and Equitable Healthcare System

To reshape the global healthcare landscape and meet the health needs of future generations, stakeholders must work together to:

- Overcome systemic barriers that hinder access to care and technological adoption.
- Implement innovative, scalable solutions that enhance healthcare efficiency and sustainability.

Prioritize equity, accessibility, and environmental sustainability in all healthcare initiatives.

By focusing on the strategic pillars of:

1. Equitable access to healthcare
2. Healthcare system transformation
3. Technology and innovation
4. Environmental sustainability

The global healthcare sector can build a future that is more resilient, inclusive, and prepared for emerging health challenges.

CASE STUDY: BUILDING RESILIENT HEALTH SYSTEMS IN THE SHADOW OF COVID-19

The COVID-19 pandemic has exposed the profound vulnerabilities in global health systems and highlighted the urgent need for increased health system resilience. With projected global output losses of US$22 trillion by 2025 and a death toll far exceeding the official 6.5 million lives, the pandemic revealed how ill-prepared the world was for such massive public-health threats. Looking ahead, the rising threats from infectious diseases, driven by factors like population growth, climate change, and human encroachment on natural habitats, pose an even greater challenge. The risk of syndemics, or the interaction of multiple diseases exacerbated by inequality, is higher than ever. This case study highlights the importance of developing resilient health systems that can prevent, prepare for, and effectively manage health emergencies. Drawing on lessons from the pandemic and other health crises, the World Bank outlines strategies for strengthening health systems worldwide, including in low-income countries.

Key Features of Resilient Health Systems
A resilient health system is defined by its ability to withstand, adapt, and recover from health emergencies.

Key characteristics of such a system include:
- **Awareness of Threats**: Proactively identifying emerging health risks.
- **Agility**: Quick adaptation to evolving health needs.
- **Absorptive Capacity**: Ability to absorb shocks without significant disruption to services.
- **Adaptability**: Modifying practices to minimize disruptions during crises.
- **Transformability**: Using lessons learned from crises to improve future responses.

Governments have two primary types of levers to build resilience: enablers and core capacities. Enablers are cross-cutting factors, including governance, financing, human resources, and innovation, while core capacities encompass health intelligence, primary healthcare (PHC) delivery, community engagement, and health supply chains.

Strategic Framework for Building Resilience
The report introduces a three-tier framework to help countries prioritize investments in health system resilience, each tier focusing on different stages of outbreak management:

Tier 1: Risk Reduction (Prevention and Community Preparedness)
- The most crucial and cost-effective layer is focused on preventive measures and community-based surveillance.
- Emphasizes strengthening primary health care (PHC)

systems and establishing community health initiatives to reduce vulnerability.

Tier 2: Detection, Containment, and Mitigation

- Focused on rapidly identifying and containing outbreaks through early detection and epidemic intelligence.
- Includes scaling up testing, isolating suspected cases, and implementing contact tracing.

Tier 3: Advanced Case Management and Surge Response

- The most expensive and least cost-effective layer, focused on managing surge capacities in secondary and tertiary hospitals during major crises.

Key Recommendations for Strengthening Health System Resilience

1. Governance and Decision-Making

- Review and strengthen decision-making processes based on evidence and real-time health data.
- Ensure clarity of roles and build a robust leadership structure, including emergency operation centers (EOCs).
- Foster multisectoral collaboration through platforms like One Health, coordinating efforts across the government and private sectors.

2. Health Workforce

- Map workforce needs and create evidence-based strategies to ensure health systems are staffed with skilled workers, especially community health workers (CHWs).
- Train and diversify the workforce to build capacity for primary healthcare and pandemic response.

3. Health Financing

- Prioritize investments in pandemic prevention, preparedness, and response (PPR), with a focus on risk-reducing measures.

- Diversify funding sources, including innovative financing mechanisms such as contingency funds, to ensure rapid access to resources during health emergencies.

4. Innovation and Technology

- Invest in agile regulatory frameworks to facilitate the rapid development and approval of new medical technologies.
- Encourage people-centered innovation, including community engagement, to ensure technologies and solutions meet local needs.
- Strengthen digital health tools and data analytics for health surveillance, epidemic intelligence, and patient care.

5. Health Service Delivery

- Strengthen primary healthcare systems, integrating public health functions to ensure continuity of care during crises.
- Develop alternative health service delivery models, such as telemedicine, to reach populations during health emergencies.

6. Risk Communication and Community Engagement

- Strengthen risk communication capacity, ensuring two-way communication with communities to build trust and address misinformation.
- Empower community engagement by involving local populations in decision-making to ensure health responses are culturally appropriate and effective.

7. Health Intelligence

- Strengthen health surveillance systems and laboratory networks to improve the speed and accuracy of outbreak detection.
- Leverage digital tools to enhance data integration and real-time monitoring of health services.

Barriers and Challenges to Health System Resilience

1. Weak Governance and Leadership: Many countries struggle with fragmented leadership structures and a lack of clarity regarding roles and responsibilities during health emergencies.

2. Insufficient Workforce Capacity: There are chronic shortages of skilled health workers, particularly in low-income countries.

3. Limited Financing: Although health resilience investments are critical, many governments face fiscal constraints, particularly during economic downturns.

4. Ineffective Health Systems: Health systems often lack the necessary infrastructure, supplies, and digital tools to manage large-scale emergencies.

5. Coordination Challenges: Poor coordination between the government, private sector, and international partners hampers effective responses.

The COVID-19 pandemic has underscored the urgency of building resilient health systems. As the world faces an increasingly complex array of health threats, countries must not delay investments in health resilience. Multisectoral collaboration, evidence-based decision-making, and community-driven innovation are essential for building systems that can prevent, respond to, and recover from health crises.

In times of economic contraction, the investment in resilient health systems should be viewed not as a luxury but as a necessity to protect both lives and economies. By building health system resilience now, nations can break the cycle of crisis-driven responses and ensure they are prepared for future challenges.

References: World Bank Group. (2024). Investing in Health System Resilience for the Anthropocene. World Bank Group.

2

THE LEADERSHIP IMPERATIVE

I n the complex and ever-evolving world of healthcare, leadership is not just a title or position—it is the driving force behind transformation. Effective healthcare leadership requires navigating intricate systems, inspiring teams, and guiding organizations through uncertainty. It shapes the direction of healthcare institutions, determines the quality of patient care, and ultimately influences population health outcomes.

As healthcare systems continue to adapt to regulatory changes, technological advancements, workforce shortages, and increasing demands for equitable access, the need for strong, capable leadership has never been greater. Healthcare leaders operate at the intersection of clinical expertise, operational efficiency, and compassionate care. Whether responding to policy reforms, integrating new technologies, or managing financial and human resources, they must align competing priorities to achieve a unified goal.

Effective leadership drives:
- Innovation is achieved by fostering a culture of continuous improvement and technological advancement.
- Collaboration is achieved by promoting synergy among healthcare professionals and stakeholders.

- Resilience is achieved by ensuring organizations can withstand and adapt to challenges.

The impact of strong leadership is evident in:

- Improved patient outcomes through informed and strategic decision-making.
- Optimized operational processes that enhance efficiency across healthcare systems.
- Adaptability allows institutions to anticipate and respond to evolving healthcare needs.

THE LEADERSHIP IMPERATIVE IN HEALTHCARE

Healthcare systems are inherently complex, shaped by:

- Multiple stakeholders with diverse interests.
- Competing demands require balanced decision-making.
- An evolving landscape influenced by regulations, technology, and patient expectations.

To navigate this complexity, healthcare leaders must address key challenges:

- **Regulatory Changes** – Adapting to evolving policies and compliance requirements while maintaining high standards of care.
- **Technological Advancements** – Integrating innovations such as electronic health records (EHRs), artificial intelligence (AI), and telemedicine into healthcare delivery.
- **Workforce Management** – Tackling staff shortages, reducing burnout, and fostering a motivated and skilled workforce.
- **Patient-Centered Care** – Ensuring that efficiency does not compromise empathy and personalized care.
- **Health Equity** – Addressing disparities in access to healthcare, particularly in underserved communities.

Healthcare leadership is not confined to executive roles. Clinicians, administrators, and policymakers all play crucial roles in shaping and improving healthcare systems.

DEFINING LEADERSHIP IN HEALTHCARE

Healthcare leadership extends beyond traditional management, demanding strategic vision, adaptability, and the ability to inspire. Unlike leaders in other industries, healthcare executives must balance efficiency with ethical considerations, patient care with financial constraints, and innovation with regulatory compliance.

Key leadership qualities include:
- **Vision** – The ability to anticipate future healthcare challenges and set a clear strategic direction.
- **Adaptability** – The flexibility to respond effectively to technological advances, policy changes, and evolving patient needs.
- **Communication** – The ability to engage and motivate diverse teams while ensuring alignment with organizational goals.
- **Empathy and Ethical Integrity** – Understanding the needs of patients, staff, and the broader community, making decisions grounded in fairness and compassion.

Clinical Leadership: Bridging Care and Strategy
While healthcare executives focus on systems, strategy, and policy, clinical leadership plays a crucial role in translating these goals into high-quality patient care. Clinical leaders—often physicians, nurses, or allied health professionals—operate at the intersection of clinical practice and organizational leadership, ensuring that decision-making aligns with both frontline realities and strategic imperatives.

Key Dimensions of Clinical Leadership:

- **Clinical Expertise with Strategic Insight**: Clinical leaders bring deep medical knowledge and use it to influence service design, quality improvement, and patient safety initiatives.
- **Quality and Safety Advocacy**: They champion evidence-based care, drive adherence to best practices, and play a pivotal role in reducing medical errors and improving outcomes.
- **Interdisciplinary Team Leadership**: Effective clinical leaders foster collaboration among diverse care teams, helping to break down silos and improve continuity of care.
- **Change Management in Clinical Settings**: They lead the implementation of innovations such as electronic health records, telemedicine, and new clinical protocols, ensuring frontline adoption and clinical alignment.
- **Mentorship and Professional Development**: Clinical leaders support continuous learning by mentoring junior staff and cultivating a culture of clinical excellence and lifelong development.

NAVIGATING THE UNIQUE CHALLENGES OF HEALTHCARE LEADERSHIP

- **Patient-Centric Decision-Making**: Unlike other industries, where profitability is a key driver, healthcare leadership prioritizes patient outcomes and safety.
- **Ethical Considerations**: Leaders frequently face complex moral dilemmas, such as allocating limited resources or addressing disparities in healthcare access.
- **Regulatory Compliance**: The sector is governed by strict policies and accreditation standards, requiring leaders to stay updated and compliant.

- **Technological Advancements**: Leaders must integrate emerging technologies, such as AI, telemedicine, and personalized medicine, while managing the associated costs and workforce training requirements.
- **Clinical Outcomes**: Have top priority and focus on the best clinical outcomes in a cost-effective manner with the best healthcare standards.

LEADERSHIP IN ACTION: LESSONS FROM THE COVID-19 PANDEMIC

The COVID-19 pandemic tested healthcare leadership in unprecedented ways. Leaders had to make swift, high-impact decisions while navigating crises, uncertainty, and resource constraints.

Key areas where strong leadership proved essential:
- **Emergency Response Coordination** – Managing surges in patient volumes and resource allocation.
- **Staff Safety and Well-Being** – Ensuring healthcare workers had access to protective equipment and mental health support.
- **Community Trust and Communication** – Keeping the public informed and reassured through transparent decision-making.

For example, many hospitals:
- Rapidly expanded telehealth services to minimize in-person visits and protect patients.
- Adjusted supply chain strategies to address shortages of medical supplies and PPE.
- Developed staff support programs to combat burnout and mental health struggles.

The pandemic highlighted the importance of agility, strategic thinking, and resilience in healthcare leadership.

OVERCOMING THE UNIQUE CHALLENGES OF HEALTHCARE LEADERSHIP: INSIGHTS FROM RATAN JALAN

Challenges in Healthcare-Specific Leadership

Healthcare leadership presents unique challenges that require a deep understanding of the complexities inherent in the industry. During an enlightening conversation with Ratan Jalan, several critical obstacles faced by leaders in healthcare were discussed, including resistance to structured change, gaps in formal leadership training, and the pressing need for accountability and transparency. These challenges highlight the nuanced nature of healthcare leadership and underscore the need for targeted strategies to address them effectively.

Resistance to Structured Change

One of the most pervasive challenges in healthcare leadership is resistance to structured change. Ratan Jalan noted that physician-owned hospitals and traditional healthcare systems are often reluctant to embrace systematic reforms. This resistance can stem from various factors, including entrenched practices, fear of losing autonomy, or skepticism about the benefits of proposed changes.

For example, implementing standardized protocols or adopting new technologies may be met with hesitation, as they require significant shifts in daily operations and decision-making processes. Overcoming this resistance necessitates a collaborative approach, where leaders actively engage stakeholders, communicate the value of change, and address concerns with empathy and evidence-based reasoning.

Leadership Training Gaps

Another key challenge identified by Ratan Jalan is the gap in formal leadership training among healthcare leaders.

Unlike industries where leadership development is systematically integrated into career progression, many healthcare leaders rise to their positions based on clinical or operational expertise rather than structured leadership education. As a result, decision-making often relies on intuition and personal experience, leading to inconsistencies in implementing change.

This lack of formal training can hinder a leader's ability to manage complex systems, navigate interpersonal dynamics, and drive large-scale transformation. Addressing this challenge requires a paradigm shift in how healthcare leadership development approaches are. Structured training programs that focus on strategic planning, communication, and change management are crucial for equipping leaders with the necessary tools to excel in their roles.

Accountability and Transparency

Accountability and transparency are critical components of effective healthcare leadership, yet they often remain underdeveloped in many systems. As Ratan Jalan highlighted, systemic processes supported by transparent data are essential for preventing recurring failures and building stakeholder trust.

For instance, leaders must establish robust mechanisms for tracking and reporting outcomes, identifying areas for improvement, and ensuring that all team members are held to consistent performance standards. Transparent data sharing fosters trust and empowers teams to collaboratively address challenges and achieve better outcomes.

Moreover, accountability must be accompanied by a culture of learning and improvement, rather than one of blame and recrimination. Leaders should encourage open dialogue about mistakes, support efforts to address root causes, and celebrate successes that result from improved processes. Ratan Jalan's insights shed light on the multifaceted challenges faced by healthcare leaders and provide a roadmap for addressing them.

By understanding and addressing resistance to change, investing in leadership development, and fostering accountability and transparency, healthcare leaders can navigate the complexities of their roles more effectively.

The challenges of healthcare leadership demand a nuanced and proactive approach. As Ratan Jalan emphasized, overcoming resistance to structured change, bridging leadership training gaps, and prioritizing accountability and transparency are essential to fostering a more effective and resilient healthcare system. By addressing these challenges head-on, leaders can pave the way for meaningful transformation, ensuring that healthcare organizations are equipped to meet the demands of an ever-evolving landscape.

THE ACTIONS OF AN EFFECTIVE LEADER

A strong healthcare leader ensures that:
- Teams are cohesive, motivated, and aligned with the organization's mission.
- Patient outcomes are prioritized, and care delivery is equitable and efficient.
- The organization is resilient and prepared for future challenges through strategic planning and innovation.

Take the example of Dr. Atul Gawande, a renowned surgeon and public health leader who has emphasized the importance of systems thinking in healthcare. By implementing checklists in surgical procedures, Dr. Gawande's leadership transformed operational workflows, reducing errors and improving patient safety. This innovation highlights how strategic, patient-centered leadership can yield measurable benefits.

Healthcare leadership is both a science and an art. It requires a blend of:
- Vision to anticipate and navigate challenges.
- Technical knowledge to make informed decisions.

- Emotional intelligence to inspire and connect with teams.
- Ethical grounding to uphold patient-centered values.

As healthcare continues to evolve, effective leadership remains the cornerstone of achieving improved health outcomes, operational excellence, and organizational sustainability.

LEADERSHIP STYLES AND THEIR IMPACT

Healthcare leadership is not a one-size-fits-all approach. Different leadership styles can significantly influence organizational culture, staff morale, and patient outcomes. Each style has distinct advantages and is suitable for specific contexts and challenges. The key lies in understanding these styles and knowing when and how to apply them effectively.

Key Leadership Styles

1. Transformational Leadership: Transformational leaders inspire and motivate teams to exceed expectations by fostering a shared vision and encouraging innovation. This style is particularly effective during periods of organizational change or when fostering a culture of continuous improvement.

- **Example**: A hospital CEO implementing digital transformation might adopt a transformational leadership approach to rally staff around the potential benefits of new technologies, such as enhanced patient care and streamlined workflows.
- **Impact**: Teams feel energized and engaged, and the organization becomes more adaptable and forward-thinking.

2. Transactional Leadership: Transactional leadership emphasizes structure, performance, and reward systems, ensuring that tasks are completed efficiently and by established protocols.

This style is best suited for highly regulated environments or situations requiring strict adherence to guidelines.

- **Example**: A nursing manager might use transactional leadership to enforce hygiene protocols during an outbreak of infections.
- **Impact**: Clear expectations and accountability reduce errors and maintain safety standards.

3. Servant Leadership: Servant leaders prioritize the needs of their teams and patients, fostering an environment of trust, collaboration, and mutual respect. This approach is efficient in patient-centered care settings.

- **Example**: A clinic director who actively listens to staff feedback and implements changes to improve their work environment demonstrates servant leadership.
- **Impact**: Staff engagement and satisfaction improve, resulting in enhanced patient care.

4. Democratic Leadership: This leadership style emphasizes collaboration and collective decision-making, making it particularly effective in multidisciplinary teams where diverse perspectives contribute to problem-solving and innovation.

- **Example**: When designing a new hospital wing, a project leader may involve physicians, nurses, and architects in the decision-making process.
- **Impact**: The result is a well-rounded plan that meets both operational needs and staff preferences, leading to higher engagement and better outcomes.

5. Autocratic Leadership: In high-stakes or emergencies, autocratic leadership provides the decisive action necessary to address immediate challenges.

- **Example**: A surgeon leading a team in the operating room often employs autocratic leadership to ensure quick, precise decisions during critical procedures.
- **Impact**: This approach ensures efficiency and control in life-threatening situations; however, if overused, it

can stifle input from others and negatively impact team morale.

Challenges and Downsides of Leadership Styles

- **Transformational Leadership** – An overemphasis on vision without attention to day-to-day operations can lead to burnout among staff.
- **Transactional Leadership** – A rigid focus on rules and rewards may stifle creativity and lead to employee disengagement if staff feel undervalued.
- **Servant Leadership** – Prioritizing others' needs over decision-making may delay critical actions or diminish authority.
- **Democratic Leadership** – Seeking team consensus can slow decision-making, particularly in urgent situations.
- **Autocratic Leadership** – Excessive control can reduce morale and lead to staff dissatisfaction if employees feel their input is consistently disregarded.

Adapting Leadership Styles to Healthcare Settings

- Autocratic leadership is crucial for making swift decisions during aublic health ccrisesor medical eemergencies
- Transformational leadership is more effective for long-term cultural and operational changes.
- Democratic leadership works well in stable settings, where empowering teams can foster innovation and engagement.

Leadership styles play a crucial role in shaping healthcare organizations. By understanding the strengths and limitations of each style, leaders can adapt to meet the unique challenges of their environment. This adaptability fosters resilience, drives innovation, and ultimately enhances the quality of care delivered to patients.

LEADERSHIP IN ACTION: INSIGHTS FROM DR. N KRISHNA REDDY

Leadership in healthcare demands a multifaceted approach, integrating personal growth, organizational management, and systemic transformation. In an engaging conversation, Dr. Krishna Reddy shared profound insights into the dynamics of effective leadership drawn from his extensive experience in healthcare.

Personal Leadership and Self-Management

At the core of effective leadership lies the ability to manage oneself. Dr. Reddy emphasized the foundational importance of self-leadership as a precursor to guiding others.

- **Foundational Importance**: Leadership begins with controlling one's emotions, thoughts, and actions. This self-discipline is a microcosm of the broader leadership journey and organizational transformation.
- **Philosophical Underpinnings**: Drawing from ancient wisdom, including the Vedas, Upanishads, and the philosophies of Socrates, Schopenhauer, and Nietzsche, Dr. Reddy underscored the importance of self-awareness and introspection for leaders.
- **Self-Reliance and Resilience**: His leadership journey has been fueled by intrinsic motivation, resilience, and adherence to personal ethics, even in the most challenging circumstances.
- **Meditation and Mindfulness**: Practices like meditation and mindfulness enhance focus and emotional regulation, equipping leaders to navigate complex and stressful environments with clarity and purpose.

Leadership Qualities and Attributes

1. Innate Leadership: Leadership often stems from a natural inclination toward improvement and learning. Dr. Reddy's experiences of taking initiative and responsibility illustrate this inherent trait.

- **Key Traits**: Accountability, transparency, and openness are the pillars of authentic leadership—a leader's ability to empower others and foster a shared sense of purpose drives collective success.

2. Empathy and Systems Thinking: Understanding diverse perspectives strengthens relationships, while systems thinking enables leaders to see interconnected patterns, supporting sustainable decision-making.

3. Delegation and Mentorship: Developing future leaders through delegation and mentorship ensures organizational sustainability and builds a culture of trust and growth.

Purpose-Driven Leadership and Organizational Alignment

- **Vision and Strategic Communication**: Leaders must articulate a clear and compelling vision, align team members, and adapt strategies while remaining true to core principles.
- **Long-Term Commitment**: Perseverance and dedication are key. Dr. Reddy shared examples of revitalizing healthcare departments, often against skepticism, as evidence of the impact of sustained effort.
- **Patience and Flexibility**: Transformation is an iterative process requiring continuous learning and adaptation. Leaders must remain committed while being open to change.

Cultivating Organizational Culture and Innovation

- **Building a Culture of Inquiry**: Encouraging teams to question norms and explore original solutions fosters innovation. Dr. Reddy likened this gradual cultural shift to the process of nation-building.
- **Collaboration and Community**: Promoting open dialogue and community-focused initiatives enhances cohesion and drives collective progress without reliance on rigid mandates.
- **Empowering Teams**: Creating a supportive environment where knowledge sharing and personal growth are prioritized fosters a resilient organization.
- **Thought Leadership**: Challenging the status quo and promoting progressive thinking leads to continuous improvement.

Experiential Learning and Practical Examples

- **Learning Through Experience**: Hands-on experiences often offer a deeper learning experience than formal education. Dr. Reddy recounted early problem-solving tendencies and their impact on his growth.
- **Leadership in Action**: Examples include managing departmental clinics, initiating clinical research programs, and creating innovative, cost-effective healthcare solutions.
- **Overcoming Challenges**: Successfully navigating complex projects demonstrates strategic thinking and resilience.

Challenges and Change Management.

- **Resistance and Adaptation**: Effective leaders recognize and address resistance to change, fostering trust and maintaining momentum to drive transformation.

- **Institutional Change**: Transformation requires robust policies and a clear vision to establish sustainable foundations.
- **Financial and Resource Management**: Effective financial oversight is crucial, particularly in resource-constrained healthcare settings.

Sustainability, Measurement, and Impact

- **Measuring Success**: True success lies in sustained impacts, improving healthcare access, or enhancing organizational efficiency. Monitoring and evaluating outcomes ensure accountability.
- **Continuous Adaptation**: Leaders must embrace diverse roles and remain lifelong learners to drive ongoing improvement. and growth
- **Long-Term Sustainability**: Aligning financial and operational strategies with the organizational vision ensures stability and independence.

Commitment to Self-Actualization and Knowledge Building.

- **Continuous Learning**: Personal development and fostering a learning culture retain talent and encourage innovation.
- **Developing Internal Expertise**: Building internal systems for knowledge sharing and participatory governance enhances organizational agility.

Building Trust and Reputation

- **Trust as a Core Value**: A reputation for integrity positions organizations as credible and reliable, fostering partnerships with governments and communities.
- **Serving True Needs**: Prioritizing service over profit builds lasting credibility and aligns efforts with meaningful societal impacts.

Connecting Leadership to Broader Change
- **Leadership Beyond Organization**: Collaborating with external partners and assessing impact within larger ecosystems magnifies a leader's influence.
- **Sustainable Transformation**: Aligning systems with long-term goals requires patience, adaptability, and a vision for collective progress.

Dr. Krishna Reddy's insights illustrate the depth and breadth of healthcare leadership. Effective leaders must navigate a complex landscape with resilience, empathy, and vision, from self-management and organizational culture to systemic transformation and societal impact. By embracing these principles, leaders can drive meaningful and sustainable change, ensuring that healthcare systems are equipped to meet future challenges.

THE LONG-TERM BENEFITS OF STRONG LEADERSHIP

Strong healthcare leadership extends beyond immediate goals, creating a foundation for sustained organizational success and enhanced patient care. Effective leaders set the tone for innovation, resilience, and a collaborative culture that drives long-term benefits.

Broad Impact on the Organization
Effective leadership fosters a thriving organizational ecosystem that supports every stakeholder.
- **Improved Patient Outcomes**: Leaders who prioritize quality care, evidence-based practices, and resource optimization achieve better clinical results and higher patient satisfaction.

  Example: A hospital system led by a visionary CEO introduced a patient-centered approach, which significantly reduced readmission rates and increased patient trust and loyalty.

- **Increased Staff Morale**: Leaders who inspire, support, and engage their teams create a workplace environment that enhances job satisfaction and productivity. This results in lower burnout rates and improved employee retention.

- **Organizational Efficiency**: Strong leadership ensures streamlined operations, optimal resource allocation, and robust decision-making processes. Over time, these efficiencies translate into cost savings and enhanced service delivery.

LEADERSHIP AS A CUSTODIAN OF CULTURE: INSIGHTS FROM COL M RAJGOPAL ON BUILDING ENDURING ORGANIZATIONS

Leadership and Organizational Culture

The relationship between leadership and organizational culture is crucial for the success and longevity of any institution. Leaders act as designers and stewards of culture, establishing the foundation for an organization's values, behaviors, and expectations. Col M Rajgopal's insights during his conversation with the author shed light on various significant elements of this connection, highlighting how leadership impact, the embedding of cultural values, and employee involvement are key factors in achieving cultural alignment and fostering organizational growth.

Leadership Influence on Culture

Leaders play a crucial role in shaping and aligning organizational culture. Col M Rajgopal emphasizes that effective leaders tackle their organizations' immediate and long-term needs. Leaders who prioritize quick wins, often termed "low-hanging fruits," enhance morale and create a foundation for

---

sizable, transformative changes. Addressing urgent matters, such as resource shortages or communication issues, can foster trust and demonstrate the leader's commitment to their team's well-being. Additionally, leaders must exemplify the cultural values they wish to instill. Their actions, decisions, and interactions serve as powerful organizational cues, signaling what is valued and expected. Through consistent and visible leadership, they build credibility and trust, key components in aligning individual and team efforts with the broader organizational mission.

Sustainability Over Personality

Col M Rajgopal emphasizes that, while a leader's influence is crucial, institutionalizing cultural values is essential for sustainability beyond the individual leader's term. Relying too heavily on a leader's personality or charisma creates vulnerabilities during leadership transitions. Organizations should instill their core values into lasting policies, systems, and practices.

This approach focuses on leaders serving as guardians of culture, promoting its development while allowing for flexibility in responding to external challenges and opportunities. Organizations can maintain continuity and resilience, regardless of the leadership in place, by fostering an environment where cultural values are deeply embedded and widely acknowledged.

To achieve this, organizations must:

- **Develop Clear Value Frameworks**: Define and communicate core principles that guide decision-making and behaviors.
- **Integrate Values into Processes**: Embed cultural values into recruitment, performance evaluations, and day-to-day operations.
- **Train Successive Leaders**: Provide future leaders with the tools and understanding needed to sustain and evolve the culture over time.

Employee Engagement: A Cornerstone of Cultural Alignment

Employee engagement plays a vital role in aligning individuals with the organizational culture. Col M Rajgopal highlights that initiatives focused on employee welfare and timely support are essential in fostering a sense of belonging. These initiatives may include health and wellness programs, skill development opportunities, and recognition for contributions. Such efforts signal to employees that they are valued and integral to the organization's success. Engaged employees are more likely to embody and effectively represent organizational values, creating a positive feedback loop that reinforces cultural alignment. Moreover, the sense of belonging cultivated through welfare programs and other engagement efforts helps bridge gaps between individual aspirations and collective goals, enabling a cohesive and collaborative workforce. Col M Rajgopal observations underscore the dynamic relationship between leadership and organizational culture. His emphasis on addressing immediate needs, institutionalizing values, and engaging employees provides a practical framework for leaders seeking to strengthen their organizational culture. By focusing on these areas, leaders can create environments where individuals thrive, teams collaborate effectively, and the organization achieves sustainable success. Leadership and organizational culture are inextricably linked, with each profoundly shaping the other. As Col M Rajgopal illustrates, leaders are not just influencers but also custodians of culture, charged with balancing immediate priorities and long-term sustainability. Leaders can align their organizational culture with strategic objectives by fostering trust, institutionalizing core values, and engaging employees, thereby ensuring resilience and driving growth. These principles form the bedrock of a thriving organization and serve as a testament to the enduring importance of effective leadership in cultivating a strong and adaptive culture.

LEADERSHIP STYLES THAT DRIVE
LONG-TERM SUCCESS

Certain leadership styles are particularly effective in creating sustainable advantages for healthcare organizations:

- **Transformational Leadership** – Inspires teams to innovate and embrace change, fostering a culture of continuous improvement.
- **Servant Leadership** – Prioritizes the needs of employees and patients, building trust and commitment within the organization.
- **Adaptive Leadership** – Equips organizations to navigate uncertainties, such as rapid technological advancements or shifts in healthcare policy.

Healthcare organizations led by these leadership styles tend to:

- Achieve better clinical and operational results.
- Retain skilled staff and attract top talent.
- Foster an environment of creativity and collaboration that drives innovation.

Few Examples:

Dr. Agnes Binagwaho (Rwanda) – Health System Transformation

- **Role**: Rwanda's Health Minister (2011–2016); Vice-Chancellor, University of Global Health Equity.
- **Context**: Post-genocide Rwanda had a $15 per capita health budget and 0.05 doctors per 1,000 people.
- **Leadership**: Binagwaho scaled immunization to 93% coverage (e.g., HPV, measles) and trained 60,000 CHWs. She introduced performance-based financing, incentivizing preventive care, and partnered with Partners In Health (PIH) for local drug distribution.
- **Impact**: Maternal mortality dropped 80%, and life expectancy rose from 49 to 69 years (1994–2020).

Dr. Devi Shetty (India) – Affordable Care Innovation

- **Role**: Founder of Narayana Health, a low-cost hospital network.
- **Context**: India's 4% GDP health spending leaves 70% of rural populations underserved.
- **Leadership**: Shetty pioneered low-cost cardiac surgery ($1,500 vs. $50,000 globally) and telehealth for rural access. He trained 10,000 nurses and technicians and localized the production of medical devices.
- **Impact**: Narayana serves 3M patients annually, with 90% paying less than $100. Telehealth reaches 500,000 rural patients.

SUSTAINING INNOVATION AND GROWTH

- **Encouraging Innovation** – Leaders who invest in research, embrace technology, and promote creative problem-solving position their organizations at the forefront of healthcare advancements.
  Example: A regional health system introduced telemedicine initiatives under a forward-thinking leader, expanding access to care for underserved populations while gaining a competitive edge in the market.
- **Fostering Organizational Resilience** – Effective leaders build systems that adapt to challenges, such as financial pressures, regulatory changes, and public health crises. This adaptability ensures long-term stability and sustainability.

LEADERSHIP, GOVERNMENT AND GOVERNANCE

From a healthcare perspective, leadership, government, and governance serve distinct yet interconnected roles. Let's highlight the basic understanding, their differences, and relevance to healthcare.

- **Leadership:** Leadership involves inspiring, guiding, and influencing individuals or teams to achieve healthcare goals, such as enhancing patient outcomes or improving operational efficiency.
- **Healthcare Context:** Leaders (e.g., hospital CEOs, chief medical officers, or nurse managers) drive organizational culture, strategic vision, and innovation. They motivate healthcare teams to adopt evidence-based practices, enhance patient care, and navigate challenges such as resource shortages or technological changes.
  Example: A hospital administrator leading the implementation of a new electronic health record (EHR) system to enhance patient data management.
  Key Traits: Vision, emotional intelligence, adaptability, and decision-making skills.
  Focus: People-centric, fostering collaboration and change within healthcare organizations.
- **Government:** Government refers to the formal authority or political system that creates and enforces laws, policies, and regulations, including those impacting healthcare.
- **Healthcare Context**: Governments (national, state, or local) fund public health programs, regulate healthcare providers, and ensure access to care (e.g., through Medicare or Medicaid in the U.S., or the NHS in the UK). They set standards for healthcare quality, safety, and equity, such as licensing requirements for medical professionals or policies on drug approvals.
  Example: A government mandates universal vaccination programs to control infectious diseases.
  Key Role: Policy-making, funding allocation, and regulatory oversight.
  Focus: Systemic, population-level healthcare delivery and public welfare.

- **Governance**: Governance refers to the framework of rules, policies, and structures that guide and monitor healthcare organizations or systems, ensuring accountability, transparency, and effectiveness.
- **Healthcare Context:** Involves boards, committees, or regulatory bodies overseeing healthcare organizations to ensure compliance with laws, ethical standards, and financial stewardship. Ensures patient safety, quality care, and risk management (e.g., hospital boards reviewing infection control protocols or financial audits).

Example: A hospital's governance board approves policies to reduce medical errors and ensure compliance with Joint Commission standards.

Key Features: Oversight, accountability, and strategic alignment with healthcare goals.

Focus: Structural and procedural, ensuring systems operate ethically and efficiently.

Key Differences in Healthcare

Aspect	Leadership	Government	Governance
Scope	Organizational or team-level	National, state, or local policy level	System or organizational oversight
Role	Inspires and drives change	Creates and enforces policies	Monitors and ensures compliance
Example	The CEO is leading a patient safety initiative	Government funding of a rural health program	Board reviewing hospital quality metrics
Focus	People and vision	Population and regulation	Systems and accountability
Healthcare Impact	Improves culture and care delivery	Shape access and public health	Ensures quality, safety, and ethics

Interconnection in Healthcare

- Leadership translates government policies and governance frameworks into actionable strategies. For instance, a hospital leader ensures staff comply with government-mandated infection control protocols.
- The government provides the legal and financial backbone for healthcare systems, setting priorities that leaders and governance bodies must align with (e.g., policies on telemedicine reimbursement).
- Governance ensures that both leadership actions and government policies are implemented effectively, holding organizations accountable for patient outcomes and the efficient use of resources.

Importance for the Future of Healthcare

- **Navigating Complexity** – As healthcare becomes increasingly complex, leadership ensures that organizations remain focused on their mission while adapting to the changing environment.
- **Driving Equity and Accessibility** – Strong leaders advocate for policies and practices that expand access to care and reduce health disparities.
- **Cultivating Future Leaders** – By mentoring and empowering others, effective leaders ensure a legacy of excellence and continuity.

The benefits of strong leadership in healthcare extend well beyond the tenure of any individual leader. Effective leadership creates an enduring impact by fostering innovation, improving outcomes, and building a resilient organizational culture. These long-term advantages enable healthcare organizations to adapt and thrive in a rapidly changing world, ultimately fulfilling their commitment to serving patients and communities. As the healthcare industry faces unprecedented challenges, the importance of cultivating strong, visionary leaders has never been more apparent.

Healthcare leadership transcends conventional management, embracing vision, resilience, and the capacity to motivate collaborative efforts for significant change.

At its core, healthcare leadership requires:

- **Visionary Thinking**: Setting a clear and compelling course for the future.
- **Empathy and Collaboration**: Building trust and working cohesively with diverse stakeholders.
- **Adaptability and Decision-Making**: Navigating challenges and opportunities with agility and clarity.
- **Empowerment and Mentorship**: Investing in people, fostering talent, and creating a sustainable legacy.

Effective leaders embody these traits, enabling their organizations to achieve critical goals such as improved patient outcomes, enhanced operational efficiency, and fostering an equitable and inclusive healthcare system.

As the healthcare industry confronts dynamic challenges, strong leadership will be indispensable. Leaders will need to adapt to:

- **Technological Disruption**: Integrating innovations like artificial intelligence and personalized medicine into everyday care.
- **Health Equity**: Addressing disparities and ensuring access to care for underserved populations.
- **Workforce Challenges**: Retaining talent and building resilient healthcare teams in a competitive and evolving landscape.

3

TOOLS AND FRAMEWORKS FOR CHANGE MANAGEMENT IN HEALTHCARE

Healthcare is an intricate field where success depends on multiple factors, including clinical expertise, patient care, operational efficiency, and financial sustainability. As healthcare systems evolve—driven by technological advancements, shifting patient needs, and policy changes—the need for structured, evidence-based approaches to managing these transitions becomes paramount. When strategically selected and properly applied, tools and frameworks serve as the backbone of transformation, guiding teams through complex challenges and ensuring successful outcomes.

The healthcare transformation journey is akin to navigating a vast, dynamic landscape. Without the right tools and frameworks, the process can become cumbersome, leading to inefficiencies, misaligned objectives, and unsatisfactory results. Conversely, well-structured approaches can streamline efforts, align cross-functional teams, and bridge the gap between clinical goals and operational realities.

Tools and frameworks act as the guiding compass in any healthcare transformation initiative. They influence how objectives are defined, processes are managed, and outcomes are measured.

The difference between success and failure often lies in their practical application. The right tools provide clarity and structure, ensuring that every team member understands their role and aligns with broader organizational goals. Conversely, poorly chosen or improperly applied frameworks can lead to delays, resource wastage, and suboptimal outcomes.

UNDERSTANDING THE COMPLEXITY OF HEALTHCARE SYSTEMS

Healthcare systems are inherently complex, involving multiple stakeholders—patients, clinicians, administrators, public health managers, and policymakers—each with unique expectations and priorities. Moreover, these systems operate within a highly regulated and ethically sensitive environment, which further complicates their operation. Successfully transforming such systems requires a combination of clinical insight, operational expertise, financial acumen, and technological understanding.

Practical tools and frameworks address this complexity by providing structured approaches to manage it. They break down significant, seemingly insurmountable problems into manageable components, allowing teams to focus on one step at a time while maintaining sight of the bigger picture.

TYPES OF TOOLS AND FRAMEWORKS FOR HEALTHCARE TRANSFORMATION

The selection of tools and frameworks largely depends on the specific goals and nature of the transformation. Below are some of the most commonly used tools and frameworks in healthcare:

1. Strategic Planning Frameworks: Tools such as SWOT Analysis (Strengths, Weaknesses, Opportunities, Threats) and the Balanced Scorecard help hospitals identify strategic priorities and measure progress across multiple dimensions.

2. Quality Improvement Frameworks: Models such as the PDSA (Plan-Do-Study-Act) cycle, Lean Methodology, and Six Sigma focus on improving efficiency, reducing waste, and ensuring consistent quality in healthcare delivery.

3. Change Management Frameworks: Successfully managing the human aspect of change is critical in any transformation initiative.

Several well-established frameworks are used in healthcare settings:

i.   **Kotter's 8-Step Process**: A structured approach for creating urgency, building coalitions, communicating vision, and anchoring change in the organization's culture.

ii.   **ADKAR Model**: Focuses on individual change with five key elements: Awareness, Desire, Knowledge, Ability, and Reinforcement.

iii.   **Kurt Lewin's 3-Step Model**: A foundational model involving three phases: Unfreeze (preparing for change), Change (implementing new processes), and Refreeze (stabilizing the organization post-change).

iv.   **NHS Change Model**: Developed by the UK's National Health Service, this model integrates leadership, stakeholder engagement, improvement methodologies, and rigorous measurement to support change at scale.

v.   **3 in a Box Model**: Emphasizes alignment between three critical stakeholders—business leadership, technology leadership, and change leadership—to ensure coordinated and sustainable transformation efforts.

vi.   **Context Model**: This model emphasizes understanding the specific organizational, cultural, and environmental contexts before implementing change. Recognizing these factors ensures that change strategies are tailored effectively to meet individual needs.

vii. **Cynefin Framework**: Developed by Dave Snowden, this framework helps leaders categorize situations into five domains—straightforward, Complicated, Complex, Chaotic, and Disorder—to determine appropriate responses. It's beneficial in healthcare for navigating complex and uncertain scenarios.

viii. **The Change Agent Model (Lawrence et al., 2006)** identifies four roles of change agents: Initiators, Implementers, Facilitators, and Recipients. Understanding these roles enables the effective orchestration of change by leveraging each participant's strengths.

ix. **Enhanced Leadership Competencies**: In an increasingly complex and fast-evolving healthcare landscape, technical expertise alone is no longer sufficient for effective leadership. Modern healthcare leaders must possess a broad spectrum of competencies that extend beyond clinical or operational knowledge. These competencies encompass emotional intelligence, resilience, adaptability, values-driven decision-making, and a deep understanding of self and others. Cultivating these traits enables leaders to navigate uncertainty, drive transformation, and foster a culture of collaboration and trust. As healthcare systems strive for sustainability and innovation, leadership competencies must evolve to reflect these multifaceted demands.

Modern healthcare leaders benefit from a diverse set of competencies:

- **Five Factor Personality Model**: Also known as the Big Five, this model outlines five key personality traits—Openness, Conscientiousness, Extraversion, Agreeableness, and Neuroticism—that influence leadership behaviors and effectiveness.
- **Schwartz's Value Model**: Identifies ten universal values that guide human behavior, providing insight

into what motivates individuals and how leaders can align organizational goals with these values.

- **Adversity Quotient (AQ) and CORE Model**: AQ measures an individual's resilience and capacity to deal with adversities.
- **The CORE** dimensions—control, ownership, reach, and endurance—offer a framework for understanding and improving one's response to challenges.
- **Emotional Intelligence (EI)** comprises self-awareness, self-regulation, motivation, empathy, and social skills. High emotional intelligence (EI) enables leaders to manage their emotions and understand those of others, fostering effective communication and team cohesion.
- **Adaptive Leadership**, introduced by Heifetz, encourages leaders to adapt to changing environments by mobilizing people to tackle tough challenges and thrive in the face of uncertainty.
- **Stewardship (ESG to ESL)**: Rajeev Peshawaria advocates for transitioning from Environmental, Social, and Governance (ESG) frameworks to Environmental, Social, and Leadership (ESL), emphasizing the role of leadership in driving sustainable and ethical practices.
- **Power of Communication**: Effective leadership hinges on clear and impactful communication. Understanding the nuances of language and its influence can enhance a leader's ability to inspire and guide teams.
- **Diverse Leadership Styles**: Healthcare organizations operate in diverse, high-stakes environments that require leaders to be agile and responsive. No single leadership style can effectively address the diverse range of challenges faced across various settings, from emergency response to long-term strategic planning. By understanding and applying a range of leadership styles,

healthcare leaders can tailor their approach to suit team dynamics, organizational culture, and situational complexity.

Whether leading through change, inspiring innovation, or stabilizing operations, adaptable leadership grounded in a solid understanding of various models is key to achieving sustained impact and high-quality care outcomes.

Understanding various leadership styles allows leaders to adapt their approach to different situations:

- **Team Leadership: Hill Model:** This model focuses on diagnosing team problems and taking appropriate action to enhance team effectiveness. It emphasizes the leader's role in monitoring and intervening as necessary.
- **Situational Leadership**: Hersey and Blanchard propose that effective leadership depends on the readiness levels of followers. Based on the situation, leaders must adapt their style, directing, coaching, supporting, or delegating.
- **Transformational Leadership: Bass & Avolio:** This approach centers on inspiring and motivating followers to exceed expectations by focusing on vision, intellectual stimulation, and individualized consideration.
- **Adaptive Leadership**: Encourages flexibility and responsiveness to change, enabling leaders to navigate complex challenges by fostering innovation and resilience.
- **VUCA Framework**: This framework addresses leadership in environments characterized by Volatility, Uncertainty, Complexity, and Ambiguity. Leaders are equipped to make decisions and guide organizations through turbulent times.
- **Technology Implementation Frameworks:** Models such as Agile and Waterfall provide a structure for

planning, execution, and iterative improvement in projects involving new technologies.

- **Regulatory and Compliance Tools**: Tools such as compliance checklists and risk assessment frameworks help hospitals meet stringent healthcare regulations, including the Health Insurance Portability and Accountability Act (HIPAA) and the General Data Protection Regulation (GDPR).

Integrating Culture Assessment into Healthcare Transformation

Culture plays a pivotal role in the success of any healthcare transformation. While strategies, tools, and frameworks provide structure, the underlying culture determines how effectively these are adopted and sustained. A culture assessment provides a structured approach to evaluating and aligning an organization's values, behaviors, and beliefs with its strategic objectives, particularly during periods of change.

Why Culture Assessment Matters in Healthcare Transformation

- **Aligns with Strategic Goals**: A misalignment between culture and strategy can hinder progress. For example, an innovation-driven hospital may struggle if its culture remains risk-averse and hierarchical. Culture assessment identifies these disconnects and provides a basis for cultural realignment.
- **Enhances Change Readiness**: Organizations that value adaptability and learning are better positioned to embrace change. Assessing culture helps leaders determine whether their teams can adapt and effectively adopt new models or technologies.
- **Improves Engagement and Retention**: A supportive, inclusive culture enhances employee satisfaction and reduces attrition. In healthcare settings where burnout is

prevalent, culture assessments identify morale issues and inform targeted interventions.

- **Promotes Ethical Practice and Accountability**: Cultures rooted in transparency and ethical behavior reduce risks of malpractice or compliance violations. Regular assessments can flag areas where organizational values are not consistently practiced.

- **Strengthens DEI and Trust**: Assessing culture through diversity, equity, and inclusion (DEI) ensures all voices are heard. It also builds trust among stakeholders when values are visibly aligned with actions.

Frameworks and Models for Culture Assessment in Healthcare

Several established models support culture assessment, each offering unique insights depending on the context:

- **Organizational Culture Assessment Instrument (OCAI)**: Based on the Competing Values Framework, this tool identifies whether a culture leans toward collaboration (Clan), innovation (Adhocracy), results (Market), or control (Hierarchy).

- **Denison Organizational Culture Model**: This model emphasizes mission, adaptability, involvement, and consistency—traits linked directly to performance.

- **Schein's Model of Culture** explores culture at three levels—visible artifacts, stated values, and unconscious assumptions—which helps understand deeper cultural dynamics.

- **Hofstede's Dimensions**: This model, particularly relevant for multicultural healthcare environments, assesses power distance, individualism, and uncertainty avoidance, among other factors.

Assessment and Change Strategies

There are two primary approaches to cultural assessment:

- **Quantitative Tools** (e.g., Safety Attitude Questionnaire) measure domains like teamwork, communication, and perceptions of management to identify areas for intervention.
- **Qualitative Frameworks** (e.g., Manchester Patient Safety Framework) focus on guided reflection, often via workshops, to foster local ownership and insight.

While both are valuable, culture is not easily manipulated. Purposeful engagement, especially in areas such as leadership, psychological safety, and learning environment, is more impactful than top-down mandates.

Steps for Conducting a Culture Assessment in a Healthcare Setting

1. **Secure Leadership Commitment**: Engage leadership early to endorse the process and commit to action based on findings.
2. **Select an Appropriate Model**: Choose based on the organizational priorities—performance, innovation, or psychological safety.
3. **Collect Data**: Use a mix of surveys (e.g., OCAI, Denison), interviews, and observations. Ensure anonymity and broad participation to gather honest feedback.
2. **Analyze and Interpret**: Quantify culture types or traits, and identify mismatches between current and desired states.
3. **Develop Action Plans**: Address cultural gaps through targeted programs, such as leadership training, diversity, equity, and inclusion (DEI) initiatives, or policy changes.

4. **Monitor Progress**: Culture evolves. Reassess periodically (e.g., every 12–18 months) to track improvements and recalibrate as needed.

Application in Healthcare Transformation

For example, assessing a hospital undergoing digital transformation may reveal a hierarchical culture resistant to change. By recognizing this early, leaders can introduce interventions to promote psychological safety, celebrate experimentation, and empower frontline teams.

Similarly, in rural health models or home healthcare initiatives, understanding local cultural dynamics, such as community trust, gender roles, and communication norms, can significantly impact the success of implementation. A culture assessment enables tailoring strategies to these nuances. Culture is the invisible yet powerful force that shapes how change is received, adopted, and sustained. Incorporating structured culture assessment into healthcare transformation initiatives ensures alignment between strategic goals and everyday behaviors. It fosters environments where innovation, inclusivity, and ethical care flourish, making transformation efforts effective and enduring.

Leadership, Balance, and Context

Evidence suggests that positive shifts in culture correlate with improved outcomes when supported by:

- Strong and visible leadership
- A psychologically safe environment where staff can speak up
- A balanced approach across cultural dimensions— innovation, accountability, participation, and performance

It's also critical to understand that cultural transformation is contingent. What works in one setting may not work in another.

Therefore, improvement efforts should be tailored to specific organizational contexts.

MEASURING CULTURE IN HEALTHCARE: LESSONS FROM THE NHS

Organizational culture is increasingly recognized as a key determinant of patient safety, staff wellbeing, and service performance. In the NHS, a series of high-profile failures—from Mid Staffordshire to Morecambe Bay—have underscored the urgent need to understand better and actively manage healthcare culture.

Current Practices in Cultural Assessment

A national survey of NHS trusts (Simpson et al., 2019) found that while most organizations are engaged in measuring culture, the approaches are fragmented, tool-dependent, and inconsistently applied. Most trusts rely on a single instrument, despite recognition that no single tool captures the full complexity of organizational culture.

The most commonly used tools include:

- **NHS Staff Survey** – Widely used to assess workforce morale, perceptions of care quality, and engagement.
- **Manchester Patient Safety Framework (MaPSaF)** – Focuses on team-based safety culture reflection.
- **Culture and Leadership Programme** – Measures and guides strategic cultural change through inclusive leadership development.
- **Safety Attitudes Questionnaire (SAQ)** – Quantifies attitudes across domains such as teamwork, stress recognition, and perceptions of management.

Despite varied satisfaction levels, many tools prioritize patient safety over the root determinants of culture, such as leadership dynamics, incivility, or accountability structures.

Emerging Gaps and Priorities

Survey respondents noted key dimensions that are often underrepresented in current tools:

- **Incivility and Bullying** – Cited by 42% of respondents as a critical but under-assessed aspect of culture.
- **Staff Morale and Whistleblowing** – Identified as areas lacking adequate measurement.
- **Leadership Inclusion** – While leadership is a well-known cultural driver, many tools fail to capture its full impact or visibility.

These findings highlight the need for a more nuanced, multi-method approach to cultural assessment that can illuminate structural and behavioral factors.

Implications for Transformation Leaders

Transformation initiatives should treat culture not merely as a variable to be "fixed," but as a co-created, evolving system shaped by interactions across all levels. Leaders must:

- Utilize multiple tools to gain a multidimensional view of culture.
- Prioritize real-time, frontline feedback mechanisms (e.g., digital apps capturing daily mood or incivility).
- View culture as both a product of individual behavior and system design.

A shift toward integrating cultural metrics with governance, staffing, and service delivery will better inform change strategies and accelerate learning across the system.

References

1. Simpson, D., Hamilton, S., McSherry, R., & McIntosh, R. (2019). *Measuring and assessing healthcare organisational culture in England's National Health Service: A snapshot of current tools and tool use.* Healthcare, 7(4), 127. https://doi.org/10.3390/healthcare7040127

2. Francis, R. (2013). *The Mid Staffordshire NHS Foundation Trust Public Inquiry.*

3. McSherry, R., & Beardsmore, E. (2017). *Healthcare workers' perceptions of organisational culture and compassionate care.* J. Res. Nurs., 22(1), 42–56.

4. Bar-David, S. (2018). *What's in an eye roll? Exploring workplace incivility in healthcare.* J. Health Policy Res., 7, 15–17.

5. Riskin, A., et al. (2015). *The impact of rudeness on medical team performance: A randomized trial.* Pediatrics, 136(3), 487–495.

Limitations of Current Culture Assessment Tools

Organizational culture remains central to healthcare transformation, yet accurately measuring it remains a persistent challenge. While numerous tools exist, most are limited in capturing deeper, intangible drivers of behavior such as trust, fear, or psychological safety.

A comprehensive umbrella review of 127 culture assessment tools (Malik et al., 2020) found that the majority were **quantitative surveys** emphasizing visible, surface-level characteristics, such as leadership practices, communication systems, and team structures. These tangible elements are undoubtedly essential, but they often overlook the underlying assumptions that shape behavior.

Tangible vs. Intangible Dimensions

Drawing on Schein's framework, the review distinguishes between:

- **Tangible dimensions**: Observable factors like policies, training, job roles, and communication infrastructure.
- **Intangible dimensions**: Deeper cultural assumptions include trust, power dynamics, blame, and moral values.

Most tools focus heavily on the former. Though critical to unlocking cultural change, the latter are far less commonly assessed. Notably, key intangible dimensions identified include:

- **Psychological safety** – Can staff speak up without fear?
- **Blame and shame** – Are errors treated as learning opportunities or personal failures?
- **Commitment and cohesion** – Do individuals feel part of a shared mission?

The review warns that relying on tools that only assess surface culture can inadvertently reinforce a belief that culture is static, technical, or mechanistic, rather than dynamic and co-created.

Implications for Practice

For transformation efforts to succeed, healthcare leaders must move beyond checklists and annual surveys. They should:

- **To surface hidden dynamics, pair quantitative tools with qualitative inquiry**, such as structured interviews, focus groups, or ethnographic observation.
- **Design-focused inquiries** should focus on trust and voice, particularly when investigating persistent resistance or low engagement.
- **Address culture as a lived experience**, not just a management metric.

Notably, the review recommends that **tangible dimensions (e.g., leadership, structures)** be treated as subtopics nested within broader **intangible themes (e.g., psychological safety, power)**—not the other way around.

TAILORING TOOLS TO THE TYPE OF PROJECT IN A HEALTHCARE SETTING

One size does not fit all in healthcare transformation. The choice of tools and frameworks should be informed by the project's scope, objectives, and the hospital's unique context. Below are key considerations:

1. Type of Project

- **Small-Scale Initiatives**: For focused improvements, such as enhancing appointment scheduling or optimizing a single department's workflow, simpler tools like PDSA (Plan-Do-Study-Act) cycles or Gantt charts may be sufficient.

- **Large-Scale Transformations**: Hospital-wide initiatives such as implementing EHR systems or redesigning patient care pathways require comprehensive frameworks like Lean Six Sigma or Kotter's 8-Step Process.

2. Hospital Size and Type

- **Small Community Hospitals**: Often operating with limited resources, these hospitals require cost-effective, easy-to-implement tools that do not demand extensive infrastructure or workforce.
- **Large Multi-Specialty Hospitals**: Larger institutions with more complex structures may require sophisticated frameworks that account for interdepartmental dependencies, compliance regulations, and broader organizational goals.

3. Resource Availability: In resource-constrained settings, tools that prioritize efficiency and minimize waste, such as Lean methodology or value-stream mapping, can help optimize existing resources without requiring significant financial investment.

4. Stakeholder Dynamics: Projects that require extensive collaboration across teams may benefit from frameworks that emphasize communication and stakeholder engagement, such as the Agile methodology, which promotes incremental progress, flexibility, and team alignment.

UNDERSTANDING CONTEXT IN HEALTHCARE TRANSFORMATION

In complex systems like healthcare, change efforts often fail not because of flawed strategy but because of poor alignment with the local context. Context models in organizational development (OD) offer structured approaches to understanding the internal and external forces that shape an organization's performance and readiness for change.

Why Context Matters: Healthcare organizations operate within dynamic environments, shaped by evolving technologies, regulatory pressures, staffing realities, and shifting patient needs. Context models help transformation leaders:

- **Diagnose barriers and enablers** to change
- **Tailor interventions** to the specific operating environment
- **Align leadership, culture, and systems** with strategic goals
- **Engage stakeholders** by mapping diverse needs and expectations

Key Context Models in Practice

- **Burke-Litwin Model**: Differentiates between transformational (e.g., leadership, mission) and transactional (e.g., policies, structure) variables. Ideal for mapping cause-effect pathways in large-scale change.
- **Weisbord's Six-Box Model**: A Simple diagnostic tool focused on purpose, structure, relationships, leadership, rewards, and mechanisms.
- **Galbraith's Star Model** emphasizes strategic alignment across five elements: strategy, structure, people, processes, and rewards.
- **McKinsey 7-S Framework**: This framework explores the interdependencies between strategy, systems, skills, staff, style, structure, and shared values.
- **Transformational Model** (Center for Organizational Design): This model offers a systems perspective, striking a balance between internal capabilities and external pressures.

Applied Tools for Context Assessment

- **Alberta Context Tool (ACT)**: This tool measures 10 modifiable context dimensions (e.g., leadership, culture, social capital, and resources) and is widely used in acute, community, and long-term care.
- **Organizational Culture Assessment Instrument (OCAI)**: Maps cultural profiles (e.g., clan, hierarchy) to guide cultural alignment.
- **Context Assessment Index (CAI)**: Quantifies barriers to implementing evidence-based practice (EBP).
- **Surveys & Focus Groups**: Capture perceptions of leadership support, morale, or readiness for change.
- **SWOT and Logic Models**: Frame internal capabilities against external pressures, proper in strategic planning.

Examples in Healthcare Settings

- **Kenya (Hospital Redesign)**: CAI revealed weak leadership and coordination. A targeted leadership program improved retention by 25% and reduced patient wait times.
- **Australia (Telemedicine Rollout)**: ACT scores indicated cultural readiness, but logistical constraints were also present. Interventions focused on time allocation and infrastructure, increasing telehealth usage by 35%.
- **Indonesia (Maternal Health)**: Community-based logic models guided midwife training and system redesign, resulting in a reduction of maternal mortality through culturally aligned interventions.

Context is not background—it is the playing field. Successful healthcare transformation requires a systematic assessment of contextual conditions. By embedding context models into strategy and implementation, leaders can enhance alignment, improve execution, and drive sustainable outcomes.

CONTEXTUAL DETERMINANTS OF ACCESS IN PRIMARY HEALTHCARE

Access to primary healthcare (PHC) is essential for achieving equity and effective management of chronic diseases. However, improving access often overlooks the contextual forces shaping service design, delivery, and responsiveness. A multi-method comparative study of primary health care (PHC) models in Australia (Ward et al., 2018) provides valuable insights for policymakers and leaders designing context-sensitive transformation strategies.

Key Contextual Influences on Access

The study evaluated four primary healthcare (PHC) models across six sites using complexity theory and Levesque's framework for healthcare access, which encompasses five dimensions: availability, affordability, acceptability, appropriateness, and approachability.

Findings revealed that **three core contextual factors consistently influenced access**:

1. **Financial Viability**: The sustainability of funding, particularly models not reliant on fee-for-service, enabled greater flexibility in providing after-hours care, outreach, or culturally tailored services.
2. **Alignment of Model Objectives**: Services with explicit mandates to serve vulnerable populations were likelier to invest in acceptability (e.g., cultural safety, interpreters, gender-sensitive practices).
3. **Relationships with Local Hospital Networks (LHNs)**: Co-location of services, shared governance, and aligned referral pathways improved both affordability and appropriateness of care.

Other important factors included workforce supply, governance stability, population health needs, and service history. Notably, smaller or newer practices often lacked the infrastructure to support more resource-intensive access improvements.

Practical Implications for Transformation Leaders

- **Design for Fit**: Interventions must be aligned with local population needs, available infrastructure, and funding mechanisms.
- **Beyond Access Metrics**: Leaders should assess deeper factors that influence implementation success, such as relationships with Local Health Networks (LHNs) and coherence of vision among staff.
- **Policy Leverage**: Structural improvements (e.g., for underserved or culturally diverse groups) often require cross-jurisdictional coordination and supportive funding frameworks.

Improving access is not only a matter of extending hours or reducing costs—it involves addressing how services are designed about their local ecosystem. In this sense, context is not merely a static background noise, but a central lever for sustainable change.

Reference: Ward, B., Lane, R., McDonald, J., Powell-Davies, G., Fuller, J., Dennis, S., Kearns, R., & Russell, G. (2018). *Context matters for primary health care access: a multi-method comparative study of contextual influences on health service access arrangements across models of primary health care.* International Journal for Equity in Health, 17, 78. https://doi.org/10.1186/s12939-018-0788-y

---

CASE STUDY: TRANSFORMING HEALTHCARE ADMINISTRATION IN MILTON MUSHEERABAD HOSPITAL

This case study examines the transformation journey of Milton Musheerabad Hospital, a 100-bed facility in Hyderabad, undertaken by an administrator tasked with revamping its operations to make it a profitable and efficient healthcare center.

The administrator addressed the challenges through strategic leadership, team motivation, and community engagement, successfully achieving the desired outcomes. In 2012, Milton Musheerabad Hospital was a struggling healthcare facility in a densely populated, low-income area of Hyderabad, India. The hospital faced numerous challenges, including financial instability, low morale among staff, and a lack of trust within the local community. The hospital's leadership was changing, and the new administrator, although experienced in rural healthcare, was formally assuming the role of hospital administrator for the first time. The initial state of the hospital revealed a dire need for intervention. Revenue was low, operations were inefficient, and patient grievances were common. The hospital lacked a cohesive strategy, and the previous administrator had failed to address underlying issues effectively. Furthermore, the community's poor perception of the hospital compounded the challenges.

Challenges Identified: Upon assuming the role, the administrator conducted an in-depth assessment of the hospital's operations, identifying five key challenges:

- **Team Motivation**: Staff members lacked accountability, direction, and morale, which hindered their productivity.
- **Space Constraints**: Inadequate infrastructure created operational inefficiencies and dissatisfaction among doctors and staff.
- **Community Engagement**: The community harbored grievances due to unaddressed concerns, poor patient interactions, and a lack of transparency.
- **Leadership Transition**: The departure of the previous administrator created uncertainty, requiring the new leader to establish authority and build trust quickly.
- **Strategic Alignment**: The hospital lacked a unified goal and clear operational strategy, which fragmented department efforts.

- **Strategic Interventions:** The administrator developed a multifaceted approach to address these challenges, focusing on team motivation, operational efficiency, and community trust-building.

Team Motivation and Realignment: Recognizing that a demotivated team was the root cause of many operational inefficiencies, the administrator took the following steps:

- **Redefining Roles and Responsibilities**: Staff members were reassigned roles that better aligned with their strengths, fostering accountability and ownership.
- **Daily Problem-Solving Walkarounds**: The administrator initiated daily rounds, personally addressing issues raised by staff and patients and demonstrating hands-on leadership.
- **Recognition and Reward Programs**: Staff members who excelled in their roles were publicly acknowledged during special events, fostering a culture of appreciation.

Infrastructure Improvements: To address space limitations, the administrator emphasized the importance of meticulous space planning and management. The installation of a new cath lab was executed smoothly, ensuring it fulfilled both functional requirements and patient needs.

- **Community Engagement:**
  - **Community Meetings**: Elders and community representatives were invited to the hospital to discuss their needs and grievances.
  - **Discount Policies**: Special discounts and offers were introduced for community members, fostering goodwill and increasing patient foot traffic.
  - **Improved Communication**: A dedicated team ensured transparent and respectful communication with patients and their families.
- **Operational Streamlining:**
  - **Collaborative Decision-Making**: Regular meetings with department heads and the newly appointed

medical director fostered a participatory approach to decision-making.

- ○ **Interdepartmental Coordination**: Team-building exercises and workshops improved coordination across the hospital's 30 departments.

Marketing and Revenue Growth: The administrator actively participated in marketing efforts, meeting with companies to resolve pending contracts and establish new partnerships. These efforts contributed to a 30-40% increase in monthly revenue within a short period.

Results

- **Increased Revenue**: Monthly revenue grew significantly, improving profitability and financial stability.
- **Enhanced Community Trust**: The community began to perceive the hospital as a reliable and compassionate healthcare provider.
- **Motivated Staff**: Team morale improved due to recognition, more evident roles, and better leadership.
- **Efficient Operations**: Departments functioned cohesively, resulting in increased patient satisfaction.

Key Learnings

The Milton Musheerabad case study highlights several important lessons in healthcare administration:

- **Trust is Foundational**: Building trust with staff and the community is essential for sustainable success.
- **Motivation Drives Results**: Empowering and recognizing employees creates a motivated workforce capable of achieving remarkable outcomes.
- **Strategic Vision is Crucial:** Clear goals and a focused strategy enable alignment and efficiency across departments.
- **Leadership Matters**: Hands-on, empathetic leadership

fosters a sense of belonging and accountability among staff.

- **Community Involvement Matters**: Recognizing and responding to community needs boosts the hospital's reputation and patient loyalty.

The administrator's experience at Milton Musheerabad Hospital demonstrates the power of strategic intervention and empathetic leadership in transforming struggling healthcare facilities. By addressing root causes, motivating the team, and engaging with the community, the hospital was turned around and positioned as a model of success within its organization.

CHANGE MANAGEMENT TOOLS AND FRAMEWORKS IN THE MILTON MUSHEERABAD HOSPITAL CASE STUDY

The transformation of Musheerabad Hospital provides a compelling example of how change management tools and frameworks can drive a successful turnaround in a challenging healthcare environment.

Applying Kotter's 8-Step Process for Leading Change

The actions taken by the hospital administrator closely align with Kotter's 8-Step Process, which focuses on creating urgency, building teams, and institutionalizing change. Here's how the framework was applied:

1. Establishing a Sense of Urgency: A rapid assessment of the hospital's dire state highlighted critical challenges, including low staff morale, financial instability, and poor community trust, which required immediate action.

2. Creating a Guiding Coalition: A leadership team was formed, comprising department heads and the newly appointed medical director. This coalition played a pivotal role in decision-making and change implementation.

3. Developing a Vision and Strategy: The vision was to transform Musheerabad Hospital into an efficient, financially stable, and community-trusted healthcare facility. The strategy focused on targeted interventions to address key challenges.

4. Communicating the Vision: Transparent communication was essential to building trust. Daily problem-solving rounds and community meetings reinforced the hospital's commitment to change.

5. Empowering Collective Action: To combat employee disengagement and operational inefficiencies, roles were redefined, interdepartmental collaboration was strengthened, and outstanding performance was recognized and rewarded.

6. Generating Short-Term Wins: Quick successes, such as the successful launch of the cath lab and immediate improvements in patient satisfaction, helped build momentum for sustained change.

7. Consolidating Gains and Driving Further Change: Regular department meetings and team-building workshops reinforced the improvements, ensuring that early successes translated into sustained long-term progress.

8. Anchoring New Approaches in the Culture: Recognition programs and participatory decision-making have become integral to the hospital's culture, fostering accountability and collaboration across teams.

Key Learnings in Change Management

- **Tailored Interventions**: The administrator customized strategies to address the hospital's unique challenges, highlighting the importance of adapting change management frameworks to the specific context and needs of the organization.
- **People-Centric Approach**: Empowering and engaging both staff and community members were central to the transformation, reinforcing the importance of stakeholder involvement in successful change initiatives.
- **Leadership as a Catalyst**: The administrator's empathetic and proactive leadership played a pivotal role

in driving change, aligning with Kotter's 8-Step Process and Lewin's Change Model, which emphasize vision, engagement, and structured implementation.

- **Sustainability Through Reinforcement**: Institutionalizing new practices ensured that the hospital could sustain its transformation over the long term, preventing regression and fostering a culture of continuous improvement.

CASE STUDY ON LEADERSHIP AND INNOVATION IN HEALTHCARE: BUILDING A HOME HEALTHCARE MODEL

The healthcare sector is constantly evolving, necessitating innovation to meet the changing needs of patients and the broader healthcare landscape. This case study examines a mission-driven initiative launched at Brooks Hospitals in 2014 to develop a Home Healthcare Model. It highlights the challenges encountered, strategies implemented, and insights gained during the journey. As a senior executive, I led the project within a resource-constrained environment, demonstrating strong leadership and collaboration to maximize the available resources from different hospital departments. Brooks Hospitals initiated a strategic visioning process to redefine its mission and long-term objectives. This involved a multi-day workshop where participants from various functions brainstormed, refined, and converted broad goals into actionable plans. One of the resultant missions was establishing a Home Healthcare business to provide essential healthcare services, like nursing care, diagnostic tests, and medication delivery, directly to patients in their homes.

Two key motivations drove the initiative:
- To provide seamless continuity of care for patients discharged from hospitals.
- To cater to the growing market demand for healthcare

services outside traditional hospital settings, aligning with global trends and patient preferences.

Leadership and Team Structure: The responsibility for implementing the Home Healthcare Model was assigned to the subject of the case study. The leadership role required:

- **Cross-sectional collaboration**: Teams from various hospital units, including operations, marketing, and clinical staff, were integrated.
- **Resource optimization**: Without any extra investment for the pilot, the team needed to utilize existing resources efficiently.
- **Priorities misaligned**: Although the leader emphasized this initiative, other stakeholders pursued conflicting operational objectives, which created hurdles for ongoing engagement.

Implementation Process

1. Baseline Study: A comprehensive baseline study was conducted to assess the needs of patients, caregivers, and healthcare providers. Inputs were gathered through interviews with doctors, nurses, and patients, focusing on:

- Post-discharge care needs.
- Home delivery of medications and diagnostic services.
- Availability of nursing and doctor visits.

2. Service Design and Pricing: Based on the findings, a service portfolio was designed, including:

- Medication delivery.
- Nursing procedures such as wound dressing and injections.
- Sample collection for diagnostics.
- Limited doctor home visits for critical cases.
- Pricing strategies were formulated to ensure affordability and competitiveness while considering resource constraints.

3. Resource Planning and Logistics: The team devised creative solutions to operationalize the model:

4. Resource utilization: Existing staff were scheduled during off-peak hours to support the pilot.

5. Logistics integration: Partnerships with courier services ensured the timely delivery of medications and samples.

6. IT and billing systems: Existing software was adapted to integrate patient records, billing, and logistics tracking.

7. Pilot Launch: The pilot was launched in a Hyderabad-based hospital to test the feasibility of the model. Key performance indicators included:

- Patient satisfaction levels.
- Operational efficiency and cost-effectiveness.
- Scalability potential for other hospital units.

Challenges: The project encountered several challenges, which were overcome with persistence and innovative thinking:

1. Cross-Functional Alignment:

- Teams from different hospital units had varying levels of commitment to the mission.
- Operational priorities often took precedence over the pilot project, resulting in delayed implementation.

2. Resource Constraints:

- Limited funding and staff availability necessitated working within existing means.
- Healthcare professionals were already stretched thin, and assigning additional responsibilities was challenging.

3. The Pace of Implementation:

- The absence of dedicated resources and delays in alignment slowed the pilot's progress.
- Gaps in continuity affected the momentum of execution.

4. Cultural and Structural Hurdles:

- Variations in operational practices across hospital units required time to harmonize efforts.

- Sustained buy-in from middle management was challenging to maintain.

Outcomes and Learnings:
- **Proof of Concept**: The model demonstrated the feasibility of delivering home healthcare services with limited resources.
- **Scalability Insights**: The pilot identified specific areas for improvement, including IT integration and workforce planning, to facilitate smoother scaling in other units.

Lessons Learned:
- **Top Management Support**: Regular reviews by senior leadership and the board provided oversight and direction, ensuring accountability and alignment.
- **Resource Creativity**: The project underscored the importance of optimizing existing resources and fostering a culture of innovation.
- **Collaboration is Key**: Successful cross-functional initiatives require clear communication, shared goals, and sustained engagement to drive results.
- **Balancing Priorities**: Managing day-to-day operations alongside innovation projects demands strategic planning and flexibility.
- **Data-Driven Decisions**: Baseline studies and pilot outcomes emphasized the importance of data in designing and refining healthcare solutions.

Broader Implications
The project demonstrated how integrating hospital, clinic, and home-based care can create a cohesive healthcare ecosystem. While this initiative faced operational and resource limitations, it highlighted the evolving role of hospitals in expanding their scope beyond traditional boundaries.

The vision of creating a connected healthcare model aligns with the future of patient-centered care, emphasizing:

- Convenience and accessibility for patients.
- Cost-effective healthcare delivery.
- Enhanced continuity of care leads to improved health outcomes.

This case study showcases a pioneering attempt to adapt to shifting market dynamics and patient needs. It reflects the complexities of innovation in resource-constrained environments and the critical role of leadership in navigating challenges. The Home Healthcare Model at Brooks Hospitals remains a testament to the organization's commitment to innovation and its ability to turn vision into a tangible reality, even under challenging circumstances.

CHANGE MANAGEMENT TOOLS AND FRAMEWORKSIN THE BROOKS HOSPITALS CASE STUDY

The development of a Home Healthcare Model at Brooks Hospitals in 2014 demonstrates how change management tools and frameworks can drive innovation in a resource-constrained environment.

The senior executive's leadership and structured approach to overcoming challenges reflect the principles of effective change management.

Applying the McKinsey 7-S Framework

The transformation aligns with the McKinsey 7-S Framework, which emphasizes the alignment of seven organizational elements to ensure successful and sustainable change:

1. Strategy: The approach aimed to expand healthcare services into patients' homes, leveraging global trends and internal resources to ensure cost-effective service delivery.

2. Structure: A temporary cross-functional team was established with clearly defined roles and responsibilities to effectively manage the pilot project.

3. Systems: Existing IT and billing systems were adapted to track patient records, logistics, and payments. Additionally, partnerships with external courier services facilitated efficient logistics for delivery.

4. Shared Values: The initiative reflected the organization's mission to provide patient-centered care, aligning with emerging trends in home-based healthcare.

5. Style: The senior executive's hands-on, collaborative leadership fostered a culture of innovation and resourcefulness within the team.

6. Staff: Existing hospital staff were creatively redeployed to support the initiative, highlighting the importance of workforce flexibility.

7. Skills: The project highlighted the need for enhanced skills in IT integration, workforce planning, and cross-functional collaboration to support future scaling efforts.

Key Learnings in Change Management:

- **Resource Optimization**: Limited resources can be overcome through creative solutions, such as leveraging off-peak staff availability and forming strategic partnerships.
- **Leadership and Collaboration**: Effective cross-functional collaboration and strong leadership are crucial for driving innovation, especially in resource-constrained environments.
- **Data-Driven Decision-Making**: Baseline studies and pilot outcomes highlight the importance of using data to inform and refine strategies.
- **Stakeholder Alignment**: Clear communication and shared goals are crucial for sustaining engagement across diverse stakeholder groups.

- **Scalability Requires Refinement**: Pilot projects provide valuable insights into areas for improvement before scaling, as evidenced by the IT and workforce challenges encountered during the project.

BUILDING SUSTAINABLE RURAL PRIMARY HEALTHCARE MODELS: A CASE STUDY

The rural healthcare landscape poses unique challenges regarding accessibility, affordability, and sustainability. Addressing these challenges requires innovative solutions catering to the specific needs of underserved communities. This documented case study examines the development of a sustainable primary healthcare model in Yavatmal, a rural town in Maharashtra, India, through a partnership-driven, technology-enabled, and community-centric approach.

The project commenced with a mandate to design and implement a sustainable healthcare model for rural areas, with a primary care focus. The initial efforts centered on a collaborative project with ITC Choupal in Yavatmal, Maharashtra, a backward linkage model in agriculture re-engineering. ITC's initiative supported farmers with technology, financing, and marketing, and envisioned adding healthcare services to its mall-like rural centers.

These centers, furnished with essential healthcare amenities such as consultation rooms, laboratories, and telemedicine systems, acted as the initial pilot site. Despite initial excitement, the program was terminated and failed to achieve the anticipated impact. Drawing insights from this experience, the team transitioned to a self-sustaining model centered on community health workers (CHWs) and localized healthcare services.

Community Health Worker (CHW) Model: The cornerstone of the new approach was the introduction of CHWs recruited from within the villages. These workers, typically women with basic education (4th–5th-grade level), were selected based on their communication skills and community acceptance.

The CHW model had three core components:

- **Basic Training**: CHWs received training in primary healthcare, including the management of common ailments such as colds, fevers, and minor injuries.
  A second phase expanded their training to include non-communicable diseases (NCDs), such as hypertension, diabetes, and high cholesterol.
- **Primary Health Centers (PHCs):** A network of PHCs served as hubs for CHWs, equipped with doctors, labs, and basic medical infrastructure. These centers were connected to a more extensive Brooks Hospital in Nagpur, ensuring 24/7 teleconsultation support for community health workers (CHWs).
- **Technology Integration**: Each CHW was equipped with a handheld biometric device powered by a Linux-based application for managing patient data. This tool supported clinical decision-making and facilitated remote consultations with doctors when necessary.

Insurance Integration: A revolutionary microinsurance product was introduced to improve healthcare affordability. For an annual premium of only ₹300, it provides coverage for consultations, medications, necessary diagnostics, and minor procedures, with a limit of ₹1,500. This insurance model was piloted with the International Labour Organization (ILO) and achieved an impressive 65% renewal rate in its first year, indicating strong acceptance and significant potential for scalability.

Community Participation and Trust Building

- **Selection of CHWs**: Village leaders, including sarpanches and elders, nominated CHW candidates.

- **Resource Contribution**: Communities provided essential infrastructure, including tables, chairs, and space in schools or Anganwadi centers, to support healthcare initiatives.
- **Recognition and Empowerment**: CHWs received public recognition for their work, fostering trust and validation from the community.

Implementation Framework
- **Training and Support**: CHWs underwent monthly training sessions at the PHC, where they gained practical skills and built confidence. Cluster coordinators provided on-ground support, ensuring consistent oversight and troubleshooting.
- **Technology Deployment**: Given the limited smartphone penetration at the time (2009–2010), the program relied on SIM-based handheld devices. These devices stored patient data, tracked treatment outcomes, and enabled seamless communication with doctors, ensuring data integrity and reducing duplication.
- **Insurance Operations**: The foundation initially managed the microinsurance scheme internally, collecting data to demonstrate its viability to formal insurance providers. Over the course of two years, partnerships with insurance companies led to the development of an industry-level product.

Key Innovations
- **Biometric Identification**: Patients received biometric cards linked to their healthcare records, ensuring accurate data tracking and streamlined services. This approach predated similar government initiatives, highlighting its pioneering nature.
- **Clinical Decision Support System (CDSS)**: The handheld devices featured a CDSS that guided

Community Health Workers (CHWs) in diagnosing and treating basic health conditions.

When symptoms exceeded their capacity, the system flagged cases for referral to a doctor.

- **Incentives and Recognition**: This program motivated CHWs through financial incentives and public acknowledgment. Honorariums and performance rewards encouraged continuous participation, while community recognition events boosted their credibility.

Challenges and Learnings

- **Acceptance of CHWs**: One of the biggest hurdles was gaining community trust in the capabilities of Community Health Workers (CHWs). Regular training, community engagement, and public recognition were instrumental in overcoming skepticism.
- **Scaling and Sustainability**: Although the pilot was successful, scaling the model required significant standardization and refinement. The project proposed offering CHWs a ₹5,000 startup loan to procure essential tools and become self-reliant.
- **Financial Limitations**: After four years, the program encountered budget issues, which led to its discontinuation. Nonetheless, the foundation established by the project provides a model for future initiatives.

Outcomes and Impact

- **Community Health Coverage**: The model served 40 villages, covering basic and secondary healthcare needs. It demonstrated that 80% of cases could be managed locally, reducing travel and treatment costs.
- **Women Empowerment**: All CHWs were women, creating employment opportunities and fostering gender empowerment in rural areas.

- **Insurance Penetration**: The microinsurance model showcased the potential for financial sustainability in rural healthcare, paving the way for future innovations.

This case study underscores the importance of integrating community participation, technology, and innovative financing to address rural healthcare challenges. While funding limitations curtailed the project's longevity, its insights into community health worker (CHW) empowerment, localized healthcare delivery, and microinsurance continue to inspire scalable models worldwide.

References:
https://www.microinsurancefacility.org/en/learning-journey/insuring-primary-care-sustainable-financing-solution-rural-primary-health/

CHANGE MANAGEMENT TOOLS AND FRAMEWORKS IN THE YAVATMAL RURAL PRIMARY HEALTHCARE MODEL CASE STUDY

The Yavatmal case study demonstrates the strategic application of change management tools and frameworks in designing, implementing, and refining a sustainable rural healthcare model.

These tools helped address key challenges, including accessibility, affordability, and sustainability in underserved rural communities. Below is an overview of the change management frameworks and tools utilized in this initiative.

Applying the ADKAR Model

The transformation aligns with the ADKAR Model, which emphasizes individual-level change as the foundation for organizational transformation.

A	**Awareness**: Community meetings and outreach programs were conducted to raise awareness about the initiative's benefits and encourage local participation.
D	**Desire**: The community's involvement in selecting Community Health Workers (CHWs) and contributing to healthcare infrastructure fostered a shared desire for the program's success.
K	**Knowledge**: Training sessions equipped CHWs with the necessary knowledge to manage common health issues and effectively use technology for healthcare delivery.
A	**Ability**: CHWs demonstrated their capability by delivering essential healthcare services locally, significantly reducing the community's dependency on distant healthcare facilities.
R	**Reinforcement**: Regular training, financial incentives, and public recognition ensured continued engagement, motivation, and retention among community health workers (CHWs).

Challenges and Lessons Learned

- **Trust Building**: Gaining community trust required consistent engagement, transparency, and recognition of CHWs' contributions.
- **Scaling and Standardization**: Although the pilot program was successful, scaling it up required standardized processes and additional funding.
- **Sustainability**: Financial limitations highlighted the need for diversified funding sources and cost-effective solutions to ensure long-term viability.

The Yavatmal healthcare model illustrates how change management tools and frameworks can effectively address complex challenges in rural healthcare. By leveraging the ADKAR Model, the initiative successfully integrated community participation, technology, and innovative financing into the healthcare system. Although funding constraints limited its longevity, the program provides valuable insights into creating scalable and sustainable rural healthcare solutions.

ENABLING COORDINATED AND INTEGRATED HEALTH SYSTEMS: A PATHWAY TO CHANGE

Transforming health systems to deliver coordinated and integrated patient care is a complex, long-term endeavor that requires multi-level action. Success depends on:

- Establishing the foundational building blocks of integrated care.
- Ensuring that these elements function cohesively to promote seamless healthcare delivery.
- Fostering shared decision-making between patients and providers.
- Building interdisciplinary teams of care professionals.
- Creating networks among care partners.
- Embedding integrated care as a standard, accepted, and legitimate practice.

Conceptualizing Change Management in Integrated Care

A successful change strategy relies on three core elements:

- **Mission and Vision** – The driving force behind the initiative.
- **Resources and Capabilities** – The tools, personnel, and financial support available.

- **External Environment** – The broader healthcare, social, and economic landscape in which the strategy operates.

For meaningful transformation, these elements must align to ensure a "strategic fit" among organizations and stakeholders.

However, integrated care does not naturally emerge within existing health and social care systems due to their historical structures and operational frameworks. Achieving sustainable change requires that integrated care systems be effectively led, managed, and nurtured.

Leaders and managers in health and social care play a pivotal role in empowering individuals at all levels to take ownership of decision-making. Experience and evidence emphasize the importance of fostering integrated care strategies from the bottom up. This approach:

- Encourages collaboration between professionals and local communities.
- Grants operational autonomy to those implementing change.
- Builds communities of practice, equipping them with the skills and support needed to collaborate effectively.

In this context, the change management process seeks to achieve three primary objectives:

- **Alignment** – Encouraging organizations to adopt integrated care as a core component of their operations.
- **Agility** – Developing systems and processes that facilitate seamless integration.
- **Attitudes** – Changing stakeholder behaviors by addressing cultural barriers through effective management practices.

NAVIGATING CHANGES IN HEALTHCARE

CASE STUDY: BUILDING A SUSTAINABLE RURAL HEALTH MODEL AT CHANAKYA FOUNDATION

The Chanakya Foundation, established by one of India's leading IT companies, aimed to address pressing challenges in rural health, education, and water access across Karnataka. The foundation operated across 200 villages in the Kodagu, Mysuru, and Chamrajnagar districts, focusing on primary health services.

However, by 2008, the foundation faced a severe financial crisis due to poor governance and limited revenue generation, threatening the sustainability of its health programs.

In response, the Brooks Hospitals Foundation took charge of Chanakya Foundation's health division with the objective of:

- Stabilizing the program.
- Boosting revenue recovery.
- Ensuring the long-term viability of primary healthcare services for rural communities.

This case study examines the tools and strategies used to revitalize the foundation's health programs, increase community involvement, and transition to a self-sustaining model.

Background and Crisis: The Chanakya Foundation had established primary healthcare centers in rural Karnataka, offering treatment for:

- Common ailments such as cough, cold, and fever.
- Chronic conditions like hypertension and diabetes.

Each village clinic was staffed by a nurse, while visiting doctors provided scheduled consultations. However, despite its scale and outreach, the financial model was unsustainable.

- For every 100 rupees spent on healthcare delivery:
- Only 18 rupees were recovered through the sale of subsidized drugs.
- The remaining 82 rupees remained unrecovered, creating a significant funding gap.

The foundation's health services relied primarily on donations and grants. However, due to governance challenges within the IT Company, a shift was required in the program's management, structure, and funding model.

Framework for Managing the Health Vertical: The first step in managing the health vertical was conducting a comprehensive assessment of existing operations. The goal was to develop a sustainable model that could be scaled and replicated in other regions.

The following key strategies and frameworks were adopted to address challenges and enhance financial viability and service quality in the healthcare centers.

Revenue, Cost, and Profit Analysis: The Revenue, Cost, and Profit (RCP) analysis was the primary tool used to assess the program's financial health. This involved a deep dive into the following areas:

- **Revenue Sources**: Identified how the foundation generated service revenue and assessed whether the pricing structure was adequate. The existing model only covered the cost of medicines but failed to recover operational expenses.

- **Cost Structure**: Analyzed the total cost of running health centers, including medical supplies, staff salaries, transportation, and infrastructure maintenance. This helped identify areas for cost optimization.

- **Profitability**: The foundation's financial sustainability depended on increasing revenue recovery and reducing dependency on donations and grants. By evaluating the balance between income and expenditure, the team outlined a path toward financial improvement.

Key Outcome:

Following the analysis, it was clear that revenue recovery needed to improve from the original 18% to a more sustainable level. By the time the program was handed over, the recovery rate had increased to around 65%, ensuring its long-term financial viability.

1. Engaging Stakeholders and Community Participation: One of the key drivers of success in rural healthcare is community involvement. The foundation already had a strong community connection, with village elders and local leaders supporting the health centers. To further strengthen this engagement, the following actions were taken:

- **Stakeholder Meetings**: Project leaders engaged with former program managers, key stakeholders, and community leaders to gather insights on the strengths and weaknesses of the existing model.

- **Volunteer and Community Leader Involvement:** The program relied on local volunteers, often elder community members, who advocated for the health centers and encouraged participation. Strengthening this volunteer network helped ensure the program remained community-driven.

- **Staff and Medical Personnel Engagement**: Staff motivation was critical to the program's success. Meetings with doctors, nurses, and coordinators provided valuable feedback on operational challenges, leading to improvements in efficiency and service delivery. Many participating doctors were retired professionals giving back to the community, so understanding their motivations helped enhance program support structures.

2. Service Portfolio Enhancement: To make the health program more comprehensive and increase its impact, the service offerings were reevaluated and expanded.

- **Chronic Disease Management:** Initially, the focus was

on common illnesses; however, the growing demand for specialized services led to the introduction of chronic disease management for conditions such as diabetes, hypertension, and hyperlipidemia (cholesterol management). New treatment protocols were developed, and staff received additional training to ensure the delivery of high-quality care for chronic conditions.

- **Preventive Care**: A preventive healthcare strategy was introduced to enhance overall health outcomes. This included diabetes and hypertension screenings as well as community health education programs. However, rural inaccessibility to diagnostic tools such as cholesterol testing kits remained a challenge.
- **Maternal and Child Health**: Addressing the needs of women and children became a priority given the rural context. New programs were introduced to improve maternal health and provide essential women's healthcare services, including sanitary napkins and hygiene education.

3. Infrastructure Development: A significant barrier to healthcare delivery in rural areas is the lack of proper diagnostic facilities. While the health centers provided primary care, they had limited diagnostic capabilities. To address this, the following solutions were implemented:

- **Diagnostic Centers**: To support complex diagnoses and higher-level care, regional diagnostic centers were established. These centers processed lab samples and offered specialized testing beyond what the primary healthcare centers could handle.
- **Mobile Healthcare Services**: To overcome geographic barriers, mobile healthcare units were introduced. These units conducted vaccination drives, provided essential health check-ups, and offered health education programs, thereby extending the reach of the health program to remote and underserved areas.

4. Monitoring and Evaluation: A robust monitoring and evaluation system was established to ensure the effectiveness of the implemented changes. This system included:

- **Data Collection**: Patient data, service utilization trends, health outcomes, and revenue recovery metrics were gathered to track program performance and inform decision-making.
- **Feedback Loops**: Regular feedback from patients, community leaders, and healthcare staff helped assess service quality and identify areas for continuous improvement.
- **Regular Assessments**: Quarterly reviews measured progress toward achieving a self-sustaining healthcare model. These reviews helped maintain financial sustainability while ensuring that the health needs of rural populations were met.

Initial Strategy: Building the Foundation of the Insurance Program

One of the early strategic initiatives was the introduction of a rural health insurance component. Drawing on prior experience with insurance data and processes, the foundation collaborated with an insurance company to design an affordable and scalable insurance model tailored to rural populations.

- **Mobile-Based Enrollment**: The foundation partnered with Vodafone to leverage mobile technology for enrollment, ensuring that even individuals with limited access to traditional enrollment methods could participate.
- **Challenges and Lessons Learned**: While the insurance program was finalized, its initial implementation faced hurdles. However, it laid the groundwork for future initiatives by highlighting the potential of integrating mobile technology into securing affordable healthcare coverage.

Integration with Hospitals: Connecting Primary and Higher-Level Care

A crucial component of the program was ensuring that rural community members had access to both primary and secondary healthcare services. The Chanakya Foundation collaborated with hospitals, notably Brooks Hospital, one of South India's leading cardiac hospitals. The goal was to provide affordable, high-quality treatment to rural residents.

- **Affordable Specialty Care**: The foundation established a referral pathway linking primary healthcare centers with secondary and tertiary hospitals. Through this partnership, community members received specialized care at significantly reduced prices.

  Example: Heart-related conditions—typically treated at tertiary Brooks Hospitals—could now be managed at a lower cost, ensuring timely interventions for critical health issues.

- **Hospital Navigation Support**: A dedicated hospital coordinator was assigned to assist rural patients requiring further treatment. Patients could call ahead, and the coordinator would:
  - Facilitate appointments.
  - Guide them through diagnostic and treatment processes.
  - Ensure seamless access to medications and follow-ups.

This structured support system minimized confusion and stress associated with hospital visits, especially for patients unfamiliar with tertiary healthcare facilities.

Strengthening Community-Based Healthcare: Training, Motivation, and Involvement

A key factor in the program's success was its focus on the people delivering healthcare services. Early in the process, a critical challenge was identified—the need to support and empower local healthcare workers, particularly nurses, who played an essential role in the care team. The foundation understood that the success of the healthcare program depended on the motivation and effectiveness of these workers. As trusted members of their communities, the nurses were deeply committed to providing the best possible care. However, they faced significant challenges, including low income, limited resources, and lack of access to digital tools that could improve their efficiency and effectiveness. To address these challenges, the foundation introduced several key strategies:

1. Technology Integration: The foundation provided smartphones to nurses, allowing them to:

- Collect and send real-time patient data to doctors and central systems.
- Communicate remotely with specialists for guidance and support with treatment.
- Maintain better contact with patients to ensure follow-ups and continuity of care.

This mobile technology integration significantly improved efficiency and care quality in rural settings.

2. Incentive Systems: A performance-based incentive model was introduced to motivate nurses and encourage the expansion of healthcare services.

- Nurses who expanded their services to nearby villages and improved regional health outcomes received a percentage of the additional revenue generated.

This system encouraged nurses to go beyond their regular duties, actively promoting better health outcomes. The financial incentives ensured long-term engagement and motivation.

3. Training and Capacity Building: Nurses received regular training on primary care protocols, including hypertension management, chronic disease care, and maternal health services.

- Training modules were customized to strengthen clinical competencies and prepare nurses for the diverse healthcare challenges they face within the community.

Additionally, a capacity-building program for doctors was implemented:

- Specialists were invited to provide on-site training to local doctors, fostering knowledge exchange.
- **Example**: A gynaecologist was brought in to train healthcare workers on maternal care, significantly enhancing the quality of women's healthcare services in rural areas.

Monitoring and Improving Healthcare Quality: As the program expanded, the foundation recognized the importance of ongoing monitoring and data collection to measure the effectiveness of healthcare services. A revamped data capture system was introduced, ensuring the right metrics were collected to assess healthcare outcomes and identify areas for improvement.

Key Initiatives in Monitoring and Evaluation:

1. Clinical Quality Indicators: Implemented standardized metrics to measure the success of treatments, early detection programs, and prevention efforts.

- **Example**: The foundation screened over 10,000 individuals for cholesterol management within one month, demonstrating significant progress in community-level chronic disease management.

2. Ongoing Training and Support:

- Established regular training mechanisms to support healthcare workers.
- Enabled nurses and doctors to contact trainers or specialists when faced with complex cases or challenges.

3. Random Audits and Reviews:

- Conducted random program audits to ensure effective implementation.
- Assessed whether quality standards were consistently met and provided corrective actions where needed.

By implementing these strategies, the foundation strengthened community-based healthcare delivery, improved service quality, and ensured that healthcare workers remained empowered and motivated to provide accessible and effective care.

The Shift in Cost Management: Reducing Dependency on Donors

In the early stages of the program, the foundation relied heavily on donor funding, with 82% of its budget coming from subsidies. However, this dependency posed a significant financial challenge, making the program unsustainable in the long term. Over time, the foundation implemented several measures to reduce reliance on donor funds and increase revenue:

Redesigning the Pricing System: One of the most critical steps was restructuring the pricing model for healthcare services. Previously, medications and treatments were provided at highly subsidized rates.

- The new approach involved redesigning healthcare packages to offer affordable yet financially sustainable pricing.
- By introducing bundled packages that included additional medications and treatments, the foundation generated more revenue from existing services while maintaining accessible prices.

Volume-Based Model: To ensure long-term sustainability, the foundation expanded healthcare access to a larger population, increasing patient volume and driving revenue through economies of scale.

- Efforts focused on improving patient engagement, ensuring follow-up care, and removing barriers to treatment access.

Cost Reduction Through Supply Chain Optimization:
The foundation optimized its supply chain management to reduce operational costs.

- By sourcing medications and supplies from new vendors offering better pricing, the foundation was able to lower costs while maintaining high-quality care standards.
- Supply deliveries were streamlined directly to rural regions, further enhancing efficiency and cost-effectiveness.

As a result of these strategies, the foundation reduced its reliance on subsidies from 82% to 35%, significantly improving financial sustainability. The combination of cost-saving measures and increased patient volume resulted in higher overall revenue, enabling the foundation to reinvest in its services and continue expanding its impact.

Engaging the Global Community: Educational Partnerships and Internships
The foundation also recognized the value of engaging the global community to enhance its programs and increase visibility. To achieve this, the Chanakya Foundation partnered with international institutions, including Harvard, Columbia, and MIT, to host internship programs.

- Interns worked on various aspects of the foundation's initiatives, including program evaluation, healthcare worker training, and educational material development.

This collaboration brought fresh perspectives to the program while fostering a culture of knowledge exchange.

- The interns contributed to program improvements while also raising awareness of the foundation's work, leading to increased support from international networks.

The Initial Challenge: The Chanakya Foundation's healthcare services were initially focused on providing free or heavily subsidized care to underserved communities, particularly in rural India. However, this financial model was unsustainable, as the foundation relied heavily on donations and fundraising efforts.

- With growing demand for services, resources were stretched thin, and the organization was operating at a financial loss.
- The primary challenge was to develop a more sustainable model that balances financial viability with continued community service.

This case study examines how a systematic approach to operations and data-driven decision-making resulted in a gradual improvement in organizational performance.

Step 1: Data-Driven Diagnosis: The initial step in effecting change involved a thorough assessment of the foundation's structure, operations, and services. The critical first 30 days of this transformation focused on analyzing key data points, including financial records, operational efficiency, and cultural dynamics within the organization.

1. Data Collection and Analysis: The foundation conducted comprehensive research into its operations, assessing:

- Healthcare service utilization to identify demand and service gaps.
- Financial status to evaluate sustainability and funding shortfalls.
- Patient satisfaction through direct feedback mechanisms.
- Surveys and stakeholder interviews, including those with nurses, patients, doctors, and community members, were crucial in identifying systemic weaknesses and opportunities for improvement.

2. Community and Staff Engagement: Beyond financial and operational factors, the foundation also examined the softer aspects of its work, such as community involvement and workforce motivation.

- Nurses often felt underappreciated, leading to dissatisfaction and high turnover rates.
- Community engagement was uneven, affecting the adoption of services and trust in healthcare delivery.

3. Stakeholder Feedback: Recognizing that both the community and healthcare providers were central to the transformation, the foundation conducted regular stakeholder meetings to align expectations and refine services.

- Nurses and healthcare workers were given a platform to voice their concerns.
- Special recognition awards were introduced to motivate and retain top-performing nurses, reinforcing their value in the workforce and fostering a culture of appreciation and trust.

Step 2: Redesigning Service Packages and Pricing - A critical turning point in the Chanakya Foundation's transformation was the restructuring of its pricing and service model. While the foundation initially provided free or heavily subsidized care, it became evident that a sustainable model was necessary to ensure long-term impact.

1. Redesigning the Pricing Model: Rather than completely overhauling the pricing structure, the foundation adopted a strategic approach:

- Service packages were redesigned to maximize value while keeping costs affordable.
- New drugs and services were introduced to enhance treatment options without significantly increasing patient expenses.

2. Maintaining Affordable Services: The foundation ensured that essential healthcare services remained accessible:

- Core services, such as consultations, were kept free, preserving access to fundamental care.
- Outpatient treatments, medications, and diagnostic services were offered at competitive yet affordable

prices, ensuring both financial sustainability and accessibility.

3. Incentivizing the Community: To expand healthcare access, the foundation implemented an incentive model for healthcare workers:

- Nurses were encouraged to extend their services beyond their assigned villages.
- Additional compensation was tied to the overall health improvements in their communities.

Step 3: Building Capacity and Competencies: Recognizing the need for skilled healthcare workers, the foundation launched extensive training programs to ensure high-quality service delivery and standardized medical care across regions.

1. Training Programs for Nurses: Specialized training programs were introduced for nurses to enhance their skills in managing hypertension, caring for chronic diseases, and implementing emergency response protocols.

- Standardized training modules were developed to ensure consistency in healthcare quality across districts.

2. Capacity Building for Doctors: Doctors participated in professional development programs, gaining expertise through collaborations with specialists.

- Training sessions were held at the foundation's Hyderabad-based hospital, ensuring continuous learning and skill development.

3. Internships and Global Partnerships: The foundation leveraged global partnerships to enhance healthcare innovation and research:

- Internship programs were established with institutions such as Harvard and the Massachusetts Institute of Technology (MIT).
- These international students contributed to research, program evaluations, and service design, bringing fresh

perspectives and credibility to the foundation's healthcare model.

- The global collaborations further strengthened the foundation's reputation, fostering long-term partnerships with international healthcare organizations.

By implementing these strategic initiatives, the Chanakya Foundation successfully improved healthcare accessibility, workforce motivation, and financial sustainability, reinforcing its commitment to transformative community healthcare.

Step 4: Monitoring and Performance Tracking: Operational excellence was at the core of the foundation's strategy. To ensure the effectiveness of the implemented changes, the foundation integrated a comprehensive performance tracking and monitoring system to measure progress and drive continuous improvement.

1. Data Collection Systems: The foundation revamped its data collection processes, ensuring that all healthcare activities—from patient consultations to drug procurement—were meticulously documented. This allowed for the development of a robust database that provided insights into:

- Operational efficiency
- Quality of patient care
- Cost management and financial sustainability

2. Key Performance Indicators (KPIs): To evaluate the effectiveness of its services, the foundation established a set of KPIs focusing on:

- Patient satisfaction levels and feedback trends.
- Treatment outcomes are used to assess the impact of healthcare interventions.
- Cost per patient to ensure financial efficiency.

3. Feedback Mechanisms: The foundation introduced structured feedback mechanisms to gather insights from patients, staff members, and community leaders.

- Regular patient surveys were conducted to assess service quality and areas for improvement.
- Frontline healthcare workers provided feedback on operational challenges, enabling timely adjustments to be made.
- Community engagement meetings ensured that local healthcare needs were continuously addressed.

Step 5: Goal-Oriented Management and Sustainability:
The foundation adopted a goal-oriented management approach, ensuring that every team member, from nurses to program coordinators, was aligned with the organization's overarching mission: achieving sustainability while providing affordable healthcare.

1. Clear Goal Orientation: Every healthcare worker, from nurses to district coordinators, was given a set of measurable goals aligned with the foundation's broader mission.

- Performance metrics were tied to incentives, including bonuses and recognition awards, to foster accountability and motivation.

2. Annual Budgeting and Planning: The foundation implemented annual budgeting and forward-planning strategies to ensure scalability and cost optimization.

- Short-term and long-term goals were clearly defined to track financial and operational progress.
- Plans focused on expanding healthcare services, increasing community engagement, and optimizing costs.

3. Cost Efficiency Strategies: The foundation reduced operational costs by procuring medicines and supplies from local vendors, thereby bypassing intermediaries to minimize distribution expenses.

- Operational efficiencies were achieved by consolidating services in strategic areas, thereby lowering overhead costs while maintaining service quality.

Step 6: Achieving Results: Over the course of three years, the Chanakya Foundation achieved remarkable milestones, transforming healthcare accessibility and financial sustainability in rural communities.

1. Financial Growth and Stability: Revenue grew from 18% in the first year to 65% by the third year, driven by increased patient volume and optimized cost structures.

- The strategic approach to cost management and scaling operations led to a significant improvement in financial health.

2. Reduced Dependency on Donors & Achieved Sustainability: The foundation successfully decreased reliance on donor subsidies, reducing dependency from 82% to 35%.

- This shift allowed the foundation to become predominantly self-sustaining, ensuring long-term impact.

3. Expanded Community Healthcare Impact: Healthcare services expanded significantly, covering over 200 villages and reaching a population of approximately one million.

- Community participation and capacity building played a crucial role in improving healthcare access and outcomes for underserved populations.

4. Increased Visibility and International Recognition: The foundation's innovative healthcare models garnered international attention, attracting a global audience of health students and researchers.

- These successes opened doors for strategic partnerships and collaborations, further strengthening its impact and sustainability.

The Importance of Initial Diagnostics and a Rapid Response: Upon joining the Chanakya Foundation, the healthcare leader identified an urgent crisis that required immediate intervention.

The first 30 days were critical for:

- Conducting a rapid assessment of existing challenges.
- Collecting data-driven insights to inform decision-making.
- Establishing rapport with key stakeholders, including healthcare workers, community leaders, and administrative teams.

This structured and systematic approach enabled a turnaround strategy that transformed the foundation's financial health, operational efficiency, and community impact, ensuring sustainable, high-quality healthcare for the long term.

Framework for Rapid Diagnostic Phase

1. Understanding the Data: A critical first step was conducting a comprehensive analysis of both quantitative (financial and operational) and qualitative (community dynamics, cultural alignment, and trust issues) data. This process, often referred to as a diagnostic assessment, should ideally be initiated immediately upon joining a new organization to ensure informed decision-making.

2. Stakeholder Mapping: Engaging both internal and external stakeholders was essential to gaining insight into the foundation's operations and challenges. The leader emphasized the importance of community involvement, particularly in rural areas, where awareness of local culture and healthcare needs significantly impacts the success of programs.

- Recognizing key figures in the community, such as nurses, local leaders, and residents, helped build relationships.
- Fostering trust within the team was a critical factor in stabilizing the foundation's operations.

3. Quick Wins: To build momentum, the leader identified quick wins that could be implemented immediately. At the Chanakya Foundation, these included:

- Awarding community nurses for their contributions.

- Aligning community events with healthcare awareness initiatives.

A well-executed rapid diagnostic phase ensures a smooth transition into the intervention phase. The following framework facilitates rapid action:

- **Data Collection Tools**: Surveys, financial records, stakeholder interviews, and feedback sessions.
- **Stakeholder Engagement Framework**: Identifying key players, their interests, and levels of influence.
- **Quick Intervention Actions**: Implementing immediate improvements to demonstrate progress (e.g., streamlining processes, recognizing staff contributions).

Building Trust and Overcoming Crisis Situations: One of the biggest challenges at the Chanakya Foundation was establishing trust among staff members, many of whom feared job losses or structural changes. The healthcare leader adopted an open communication approach, addressing concerns directly and aligning the team with the organization's long-term goals.

Leadership Tools for Trust-Building

- **Transparency**: Communicating organizational goals and expected outcomes. Emphasizing that staff positions would be retained while improving efficiency.
- **Engagement and Recognition**: Publicly recognizing staff contributions through community appreciation programs for nurses, enhancing morale, and aligning employee efforts with the organization's objectives.
- **Consistent Action**: Ensuring that organizational actions matched stated values to build credibility.
- Demonstrating commitment by following through on promises to employees and the community.

Trust-Building Frameworks for Healthcare Organizations:

- **Trust-Building Matrix**: Mapping trust levels across teams and stakeholders, then implementing a strategic plan to address gaps.
- **Transparency Protocol**: Holding regular town halls, establishing direct communication channels, and maintaining open feedback mechanisms to enhance trust and internal transparency.
- **Recognition Program**: Implementing formal recognition initiatives, such as awards or acknowledgment ceremonies, to appreciate community contributions and employee efforts.

Process Refinement and Long-Term Strategy Development: Following the completion of the diagnostic phase and the establishment of trust, the next step was to develop long-term strategies that ensured sustainability and growth. At the Chanakya Foundation, the focus shifted toward incremental improvements, particularly in revenue generation, to reduce reliance on donations.

Strategic Framework for Long-Term Sustainability

i. Revenue Alignment: The primary objective was to recover operational costs through service charges rather than relying solely on external donations.

- Redesigned pricing and services to achieve financial sustainability while maintaining affordable healthcare access.

ii. Resource Allocation and Efficiency: Optimizing operational efficiency by reducing inefficiencies in care delivery.

- Reorganizing village outreach programs to improve resource utilization.

Key Frameworks for Sustainability:

- **Financial Sustainability Model**: Transitioning from donation-dependent funding to self-sustaining revenue models and implementing service-based income streams to cover operational expenses.
- **Operational Efficiency Framework**: Conducting regular process audits to evaluate staffing levels, resource utilization, and service delivery models, and streamlining operations to reduce waste and optimize workflow.

ENGAGING WITH COMMUNITY AND RURAL DEVELOPMENT

A core component of the leader's work at Chanakya Foundation was integrating healthcare with broader rural development efforts.

By collaborating with local community groups, religious organizations, and women's groups, the leader developed a holistic approach that combined treatment, preventive care, and social engagement.

This multifaceted engagement strategy reinforced healthcare sustainability, strengthened community trust, and ensured a lasting impact on healthcare in rural areas.

Community Engagement and Development Tools

- **Community Health Programs**: The leader introduced preventive healthcare initiatives, such as screening and health education programs, tailored for rural communities.
- **Building Collaborative Networks:** Collaboration with rural development centers, religious organizations, and local community groups helped leverage resources and expand the reach of healthcare initiatives.

- **Telemedicine and Virtual Care**: To bridge the gap between urban and rural healthcare, the leader explored telemedicine and virtual care models, providing remote consultations and improving access to specialized care.

Scalable Healthcare Engagement Models

These community health engagement models can be replicated in various healthcare settings to develop more connected service delivery systems:

- **Community Health Partnership Framework**: Establishing collaborations with local organizations to strengthen healthcare service delivery.
- **Telehealth Integration Plan**: Implementing telemedicine services to extend healthcare reach and improve access for underserved populations.

For organizations seeking to expand their service offerings, the following models provide scalable solutions for rural healthcare integration:

- **Rural Healthcare Model**: A blueprint for integrating urban healthcare systems with rural communities through strategic partnerships and service expansions.
- **Telemedicine Framework**: A structured approach to scaling telemedicine services to increase access to specialized care in rural or underserved areas.

Results and Outcomes

- **Revenue Recovery**: The revenue recovery rate increased from 18% to 65%, moving the program toward financial sustainability.
- **Expanded Services**: The program evolved into a comprehensive healthcare model, incorporating chronic disease management, preventive care, maternal health services, diagnostic centers, and mobile healthcare services, enhancing the quality and reach of care.

- **Enhanced Community Involvement**: Active community participation and volunteer networks led to increased program utilization and stronger patient engagement.

Sustainability: Through improved revenue models, expanded service offerings, and optimized operations, the Chanakya Foundation's healthcare initiative became sustainable and scalable, positioning it for replication in other rural regions.

BROADER APPLICABILITY OF THESE FRAMEWORKS

The diagnostic assessments, trust-building strategies, financial sustainability models, and rural healthcare integration tools employed in this case study provide a structured approach that can be applied across various healthcare organizations, ranging from rural health foundations to large commercial healthcare groups.

These strategic principles enable healthcare leaders to:

- Manage change effectively
- Enhance operational efficiency
- Strengthen community engagement
- Ensure long-term healthcare sustainability

As the healthcare landscape continues to evolve, these frameworks offer valuable guidance for navigating transformation, enhancing patient care, and promoting resilience within healthcare organizations.

Challenges in Applying Tools and Frameworks

- **Resistance to Change**: Healthcare professionals may hesitate to adopt new processes, especially if they perceive them as disruptive or unnecessary for patient care.
- **Resource Limitations**: Many healthcare organizations operate within restricted budgets,

making it difficult to invest in training, technology, or additional resources for successful framework implementation.

- **Complexity of Measurement**: Unlike other industries where success metrics are clear, healthcare transformation often involves subjective factors, such as patient satisfaction and improvements in quality of life, which are more challenging to quantify.
- **Alignment Across Teams**: Maintaining cross-functional team alignment with a shared vision is challenging, especially in large, multi-disciplinary healthcare organizations with diverse operational priorities.

Despite these challenges, the importance of using practical tools and frameworks in healthcare change management cannot be overstated.

- They provide structure, clarity, and direction for navigating complex healthcare systems.
- They help tailor transformation strategies to align with organizational needs and goals.
- They empower healthcare leaders to implement sustainable change while enhancing patient outcomes.

By adopting the right frameworks and tailoring them to address their unique challenges, healthcare leaders can drive meaningful and lasting transformation, ultimately enhancing both patient care and organizational performance.

CASE STUDY: TRANSFORMING GANDHI HOSPITAL, JABALPUR THROUGH A JOINT VENTURE AND STRATEGIC PROJECT MANAGEMENT

Gandhi Hospital, Jabalpur, initially a 50-bed facility, underwent a significant transformation into a 200-bed hospital through a joint venture with Brooks Hospitals in 2007. This case study examines the strategic project management behind this expansion, the challenges encountered, and the key decisions that contributed to the project's successful completion.

The project necessitated significant infrastructure upgrades and a cultural and operational transformation as it transitioned from a family-owned operation to a part of a larger corporate healthcare group.

Background: Jabalpur, located in the Indian state of Madhya Pradesh, has undergone substantial changes since 2007. At that time, the city had limited infrastructure and connectivity, making it an unconventional choice for large-scale hospital projects. The hospital was initially run by Dr. Ramesh Sen, a renowned general surgeon, and his family. However, as the demand for healthcare services grew, the family recognized the need for additional capital and expertise to expand their facility and improve the quality of care. In 2007, Brooks Hospitals entered into a joint venture with the Dr. Ramesh Sen family to modernize and expand Gandhi Hospital, increasing its capacity from 50 to 200 beds. The expansion aimed to address the city's growing healthcare needs and establish Gandhi Hospital as a leading healthcare facility in the region. The collaboration brought together Brooks Hospitals' experience managing extensive healthcare facilities and the Sen family's local knowledge and legacy in healthcare provision.

The Challenge: The primary challenge of this project was integrating two different organizational cultures and executing the expansion in a region with limited infrastructure. Jabalpur was not yet fully urbanized, and the city lacked basic amenities, including reliable transportation and a well-developed road network.

Additionally, the project involved complex technical requirements such as installing a Cath lab, the first of its kind in Jabalpur, and state-of-the-art medical equipment.

The construction was a "brownfield" project—working with an existing hospital facility to expand and upgrade rather than starting from scratch. This posed several unique difficulties, including managing ongoing operations at the hospital while construction was underway. Furthermore, the project had to be executed within a strict timeline and budget, with the expectation that the hospital would be operational and ready for inauguration by 2008.

Key Project Management Strategies:

- **Understanding Stakeholder Needs and Aligning Goals**

The project team recognized that successful execution required understanding the stakeholders' perspectives and aligning their goals. The family-run hospital had a strong legacy and unique operational style, which must be considered when planning and implementing the expansion.

This required continuous communication with Dr. Sen's and his family to understand their hospital's vision and expectations for the expansion.

A critical aspect of the alignment was understanding Dr. Sen's family's desire for rapid results. While Brooks Hospitals brought in expertise, capital, and technology, the family was heavily involved in decisions related to the design and execution of the project. The challenge was to balance the desire for speed with ensuring the highest standards of quality and patient care.

- **Cultural Sensitivity and Relationship Building**

One of the most significant challenges encountered was the cultural gap between Brooks Hospitals' professional management approach and the more family-centric, less formal operations of Dr. Sen's family. The hospital administrators and family members had limited exposure to corporate management practices. Brooks Hospitals had to adopt a more flexible, coaching, and participatory approach to help them understand the intricacies of professional healthcare management.

The project manager spent significant time with the family to understand their concerns and foster trust, which was crucial for ensuring smooth collaboration. A key success factor was the adaptability and flexibility of Brooks Hospitals' team. Instead of imposing external management practices, they worked closely with the family to guide them through the process, adapting their methods to the family's cultural and operational context. This approach minimized friction and helped build trust over time.

- **Effective Project Execution**

The project's success relied heavily on effective project management techniques, especially in coordinating the various contractors, departments, and stakeholders. The expansion involved complex logistics, including the installation of high-end biomedical equipment and specialized infrastructure, such as HVAC systems. This required careful planning and coordination with local contractors and suppliers. One of the key lessons from this case was the importance of precise alignment between the different teams involved in the project. The project manager ensured that all stakeholders, from construction teams to medical equipment suppliers, were aligned with the overall goals and timelines. This required consistent monitoring and daily updates to track progress and resolve issues in real-time. The project encountered numerous challenges, including delays in equipment delivery and logistical difficulties in transporting materials to Jabalpur. One major hurdle was with the HVAC system, which was crucial for the hospital's operations. The vendor faced delays, but the project manager escalated the issue and worked closely with the regional head to resolve the situation. This level of proactive management was crucial in ensuring that critical systems, such as HVAC, were installed on time.

- **Adaptation to Local Context**

Another central learning from this project was the importance of adapting to the local context. Jabalpur was an emerging city with a predominantly rural population. Many hospital staff and patients come from tribal or less urbanized areas, so the project manager must be mindful of their needs and preferences. The language barrier, varying levels of education, and cultural norms required a more hands-on approach, with continuous monitoring and coaching to ensure that all team members were on track and that the project was progressing smoothly. Furthermore, the project manager worked closely with the local community to understand their healthcare needs, particularly regarding infrastructure like the general ward. Adjustments were made to the hospital design based on local requirements, including increasing the number of general ward beds to better cater to the community's needs.

Outcome and Impact:

Despite the numerous challenges, Gandhi Hospital successfully launched the expanded facility in 2008, two weeks ahead of schedule. Chief Minister Vikram Aditya inaugurated the hospital, quickly becoming one of the region's leading healthcare facilities. The expansion included the introduction of advanced medical technologies, such as the cath lab, as well as an expanded intensive care unit (ICU) and general wards.

Today, Gandhi Hospital has evolved into a 400-bed facility, providing world-class healthcare services to the residents of Jabalpur and its surrounding areas. The project successfully achieved its construction goals on time and within budget, laying the foundation for a sustainable, high-quality healthcare system that serves a growing and diverse population.

The transformation of Gandhi Hospital demonstrates the power of strategic project management, cultural sensitivity, and stakeholder engagement in healthcare projects. Brooks Hospitals successfully expanded Gandhi Hospital into a leading healthcare provider in the region by carefully navigating the complexities of a joint venture, aligning stakeholder expectations, and adapting to the local context.

This case study underscores the importance of flexibility, relationship-building, and proactive problem-solving in successfully executing complex healthcare projects.

CHALLENGES IN TRANSFORMING GANDHI HOSPITAL, JABALPUR: A CHANGE MANAGEMENT PERSPECTIVE

The Gandhi Hospital project, which involved expanding a 50-bed hospital into a 200-bed facility, encountered significant challenges due to the transition from a family-run institution to a corporate-managed hospital under a joint venture with Brooks Hospitals. These challenges were rooted in cultural shifts, stakeholder alignment, operational changes, and the need to balance family involvement with professionalism.

1. Cultural Resistance to Change: The hospital was initially managed by a family, operating with a relationship-driven, informal style rather than structured systems and processes. The transition to a corporate governance model under Brooks Hospitals required a shift toward formalized protocols, reporting structures, and performance-based metrics.

- The family members involved in hospital operations, many of whom lacked professional training, struggled to align with the structured, process-driven approach that Brooks Hospitals intended to introduce.
- The resistance was most substantial from those accustomed to running operations informally, as they found corporate-style management rigid and feared losing control over daily decision-making.

2. Managing Stakeholder Expectations: The promoter family had high expectations for the hospital's design and operations, wanting significant control over its execution. However, Brooks Hospitals needed to maintain corporate standards, clinical protocols, and a scalable, sustainable model.

- Balancing the family's vision with Brooks Hospitals' structured approach required continuous negotiation, trust-building, and conflict resolution.
- The project management team had to ensure that the hospital's transformation aligned with corporate healthcare standards without alienating the family's influence.

3. Changing the Operational Approach: The hospital had been operating with minimal formalized processes. With the joint venture, new systems for hospital administration, clinical protocols, training, and IT infrastructure had to be introduced.

- Resistance from existing staff, including doctors, nurses, and administrative personnel, stemmed from unfamiliarity with standardized procedures. Many were accustomed to making independent decisions rather than following structured workflows and accountability measures.
- Implementing new hospital management software, digital patient records, and protocol-driven medical procedures required extensive training, clear communication, and hands-on leadership to help staff adapt.

4. Balancing Professionalism and Family Involvement: The head surgeon and key family members maintained significant influence over hospital operations, creating tension between their personalized, ad-hoc decision-making style and Brooks Hospital's professional, process-driven approach.

- The challenge was to ensure the family's continued involvement without undermining the need for structured governance and operational efficiency.
- The project management team worked closely with the family to integrate their vision while implementing necessary organizational changes, ensuring a balanced transition that honored the family's legacy while preparing the hospital for scalable growth.

- The transformation of Gandhi Hospital illustrates the challenges of merging traditional, family-run healthcare institutions with corporate healthcare management models. Successfully navigating this transition required cultural sensitivity, structured change management strategies, and strong leadership to align stakeholders while maintaining operational excellence.

5. Infrastructure and Resource Management: In 2007, Jabalpur was less developed in terms of infrastructure and connectivity compared to its current state. This posed challenges in sourcing medical materials and equipment, transporting goods, and ensuring timely project completion. The hospital's remote location made it challenging to procure specialized medical equipment, such as the cath lab, which had to be sourced from other cities.

- Since the project involved expanding a brownfield hospital, it required working with existing infrastructure while incorporating new facilities. Unlike a greenfield project, modifications to the existing hospital structure had to be carefully planned to avoid disruptions to ongoing hospital operations.

6. Communication and Collaboration Across Teams: Effective communication was critical in managing this large-scale hospital expansion. The project involved multiple stakeholders, including Brooks Hospitals, the local administration, the hospital's operational team, and contractors.

- The hospital's family owners were deeply involved in decision-making, which sometimes created communication gaps between them and the professional hospital management team.

- Regular progress updates were provided; however, challenges arose in aligning the expectations of different stakeholders, particularly when project delays occurred. For example, the procurement and installation of HVAC systems encountered setbacks, necessitating prompt issue resolution and effective escalation management to prevent more significant disruptions.

7. **Adapting to Local Context and Needs:** Jabalpur's population, including many from tribal areas, had unique healthcare expectations and specific needs.

   The hospital staff had to be trained to accommodate linguistic, cultural, and socio-economic differences in patient care.

- Brooks Hospitals had to adapt its clinical and operational practices to serve diverse patient demographics, including working-class communities from surrounding rural areas.

8. Ensuring Timely Completion and Managing Delays: Despite various challenges, the hospital expansion was completed on time—in fact, it was launched two weeks ahead of schedule. However, delays were a constant risk, whether due to transportation issues, material shortages, or vendor-related setbacks.

- Change management in this context required adaptability, quick decision-making, and problem-solving to prevent setbacks from derailing the project.
- For instance, when flooring materials were delayed, the project team acted swiftly, mobilizing additional resources to ensure completion in time for the Chief Minister's inauguration event.

The Project Required:
- Navigating cultural resistance within a family-run hospital transitioning to corporate governance.
- Ensuring seamless communication and collaboration across diverse stakeholders.
- Adapting operations to meet the needs of Raipur's diverse patient population.
- Strategically managing infrastructure to prevent disruptions to hospital operations.

- Proactively addressing supply chain and logistical hurdles.

Applying Change Management Strategies to Overcome These Challenges

Structured change management strategies could have further optimized the project by reducing resistance, improving stakeholder alignment, and ensuring smoother transitions.

1. Cultural Resistance to Change

- **Solution: Clear Vision and Communication**
  - Change management frameworks, such as Kotter's 8-Step Model, emphasize the importance of establishing a clear vision and communicating changes regularly to gain stakeholder buy-in.
  - Frequent town halls, feedback sessions, and structured transition planning could have helped the hospital staff and family owners adapt to corporate governance more effectively.

2. Managing Stakeholder Expectations

- **Solution: Stakeholder Mapping and Engagement**
  - Stakeholder mapping helps identify all key players (family owners, doctors, administrators, vendors, and local government).
  - Conducting regular alignment meetings with hospital promoters and Brooks Hospitals' leadership would have ensured clear expectations, reduced conflicts, and fostered trust in the decision-making process.
  - By applying structured change management strategies, healthcare leaders can mitigate resistance, align stakeholder expectations, and ensure the seamless execution of large-scale projects.

3. Changing the Operational Approach
- **Solution: Training and Capability Building**
  - A well-designed training program is essential for overcoming resistance to new operational approaches.
  - A structured training plan should have been implemented early in the transition to educate hospital staff, doctors, and management about the new systems, processes, and technologies.
  - In addition to formal training, ongoing support mechanisms such as mentoring, peer learning sessions, and hands-on workshops could have ensured that staff felt supported throughout the transition. This approach would reduce anxiety and increase confidence in using new systems.
  - Implementing incremental change, rather than an abrupt overhaul, could have helped ease resistance by introducing minor, manageable improvements rather than overwhelming operational shifts.

4. Infrastructure and Resource Management
- **Solution: Project Management Best Practices**
  - Applying project management methodologies such as Agile or Lean Six Sigma could have optimized resource allocation, managed logistical hurdles, and improved overall efficiency.
  - These methodologies emphasize iterative improvements, continuous feedback, and structured workflows, which could have helped mitigate supply chain disruptions and infrastructure bottlenecks.
  - Proactive supply chain planning and risk assessment frameworks would have ensured that critical medical equipment and construction materials were procured and deployed efficiently.

5. Adapting to Local Context and Needs
- **Solution: Cultural Sensitivity and Local Adaptation**
  - A successful change management strategy in healthcare must be deeply attuned to the cultural, social, and economic realities of the patients and community it serves.
  - The transition process should have incorporated local perspectives, ensuring that staff training, patient communication strategies, and hospital workflows aligned with community expectations.
  - Community engagement programs, feedback sessions, and localized training approaches could have bridged the gaps between new corporate practices and traditional ways of working.

REVITALIZING HEALTHCARE OPERATIONS : ALWYN HOSPITAL – A CASE STUDY OF TOOLS AND FRAMEWORKS

Transforming an underperforming hospital into a sustainable, profitable entity is an intricate journey. This case study examines the methodology employed by a hospital administrator who successfully transformed a multi-specialty hospital in Kochi. By leveraging diagnostic tools, stakeholder engagement, and structured frameworks, this case study provides insights into the practical application of leadership in healthcare.

Background: Alwyn Hospital began as a charitable oncology center founded by philanthropists from Kochi. Initially operated on leased premises, it served the community by providing affordable cancer care.

Over time, the organization invested nearly ₹ 200 crores to build a multi-specialty hospital, broadening its impact while ensuring financial sustainability. However, the transition from charity to sustainability proved challenging.

The new hospital incurred continuous financial losses, raising questions about its viability. Let's outline the systematic approach adopted by the hospital's new leadership to reverse this trend.

PHASE 1: DIAGNOSIS AND INITIAL ASSESSMENT - Upon assuming leadership in May 2016, the new Hospital Administrator began by conducting a comprehensive diagnosis of the hospital's financial, operational, and cultural health.

The key activities during this phase included:

i. Profit and Loss Analysis

- A detailed review of the hospital's profit and loss (P&L) statements over the last three to five years helped identify trends in revenue, costs, and profitability.
- Emphasis was placed on understanding EBITDA (Earnings Before Interest, Taxes, Depreciation, and Amortization) and its contributing factors.

ii. Contribution Analysis

- Revenue was analyzed against variable costs to calculate contribution margins.
- Interest, depreciation, and profitability patterns provided a foundation for understanding financial challenges.

iii. Volume Study

- Historical data on outpatient (OPD) and inpatient department volumes were scrutinized.
- The performance of each specialty was analyzed to identify its strengths and areas that require attention.

iv. Stakeholder Engagement

- Initial meetings with doctors and departmental heads helped uncover operational bottlenecks and service gaps.
- One-on-one sessions with doctors provided valuable insights into their perspectives, concerns, and ideas for improvement.

PHASE 2: INTERNAL AND EXTERNAL ECOSYSTEM ANALYSIS - The second phase involved a deeper exploration of internal operations and external market dynamics.

i. Departmental Analysis
- Interactions with key departments such as HR, IT, operations, nursing, and supply chain management (SCM) helped uncover challenges and inefficiencies.
- Regular senior leadership meetings established a culture of open communication and collaboration.

ii. Cultural Assessment
- Kochi's unique societal culture presented both opportunities and challenges.
- The local population's high expectations and preference for personalized care influenced satisfaction levels.

iii. Market Ecosystem Study
- A thorough examination of competitors, market practices, and patient demographics provided a strategic view of the hospital's positioning.
- Visits to local clinics, nursing homes, and other healthcare facilities provided valuable insights into external perceptions of the hospital.

iv. Stakeholder Relationships
- Key stakeholders, including regulatory bodies, charitable committees, and corporate clients, were engaged to rebuild trust and address unresolved issues.
- For instance, addressing delayed pharmacy regulations and kidney transplant approvals became immediate priorities.

Frameworks Utilized: The administrator utilized several frameworks to guide the analysis and strategy development:

a. PESTEL Analysis
- This framework helped assess external factors, including Political, Economic, Social, Technological,

Environmental, and Legal elements, that impact the hospital.

- The hospital could align its operations with external demands by identifying gaps in these areas.

b. SWOT Analysis: A SWOT (Strengths, Weaknesses, Opportunities, and Threats) analysis was conducted for the hospital, providing a comprehensive view of its internal and external environment.

c. GAP Analysis: A detailed gap analysis revealed over 200 actionable points, encompassing financial, operational, and stakeholder-related challenges.

PHASE 3: ENGAGING STAKEHOLDERS - Effective stakeholder management emerged as a cornerstone of the turnaround strategy. Key initiatives included:

i. Doctors and Medical Staff

- One-on-one meetings were held with all doctors to understand their challenges and align them with the hospital's goals.
- Doctors from outside the hospital were also consulted to gather unbiased feedback.

ii. Departments and Teams

- Each department was evaluated for its operational effectiveness, with special attention given to revenue cycle management (RCM) and supply chain management (SCM).
- Training programs were introduced to upskill staff and address service delivery gaps.

iii. Regulatory Bodies

- The hospital strengthened its relationships with health regulators, ensuring compliance and smoother approval processes.

iv. Charity and Community

- Regular interactions with the charitable committee

helped rebuild trust and honor commitments to the community.
- The hospital also worked to align its services with the cultural expectations of Kochin society.

v. Market Perception
- External doctors and administrators were engaged to address concerns about competition and collaboration.
- The hospital repositioned itself as a partner rather than a competitor in the local healthcare ecosystem.

PHASE 4: IMPLEMENTING CHANGE – Based on the insights gathered during diagnosis and analysis, a strategic roadmap was implemented:

i. Operational Improvements
- Streamlined processes in key areas such as billing, appointments, and emergency services.
- Enhanced patient experience through better queuing systems, trained staff, and improved communication.

ii. Financial Restructuring
- Cost-cutting measures were introduced, focusing on optimizing variable costs without compromising the quality of care.
- New revenue streams were identified, including corporate partnerships and specialized services.

iii. Cultural Transformation
- Efforts were made to align staff behavior with local cultural norms, emphasizing empathy and personalized care.
- Community outreach programs helped build goodwill and trust.

iv. Marketing and Branding
- A dual approach to branding and sales ensured greater visibility and improved patient acquisition.
- Focused campaigns highlighted the hospital's specialties and community contributions.

Results and Impact

- **Financial Turnaround**: Hospital Administrator joined in May 2016, and the hospital was operating at a loss. By June 2016, it achieved profitability, maintaining a 15-18% profit margin until February 2018. This turnaround marked the highest profitability within the Alwyn Group during that period.

- **Team Development**: A strong, cohesive team was established, with a pipeline of future leaders poised to assume higher organizational responsibilities.

- **Favorable Ecosystem**: Internal morale improved, and external perceptions began to shift. The hospital established itself as a trusted and respected institution in the region.

- **Sustainable Growth**: The strategic planning and expansion efforts, which focus on local and regional markets, lay the groundwork for long-term growth. Long-term initiatives, such as expanding services to neighboring states and developing future leaders, ensured sustained growth and resilience.

- **Enhanced Reputation**: Strategic interventions transformed the hospital's external image. From hosting the first CII conference in the Western region to fostering positive relationships with government officials, the hospital positioned itself as a key stakeholder in the regional healthcare ecosystem.

EXPLORING THE PHASES IN DETAIL

A strong organizational culture is a critical determinant of success. In a healthcare setting, culture is shaped by daily departmental meetings, planning sessions, and routine interactions. These foundational elements ensure goal alignment and operational efficiency.

Key Cultural Elements:
 1. Team Structure and Motivation:
- Understanding the existing team hierarchy and motivational factors is crucial.
- Identifying competency gaps and resource requirements helps build a cohesive and high-performing team.

2. Integration of Diverse Teams: In multicultural and mixed-skill environments, fostering team cohesion is crucial.

For example, in the Kochi hospital setting, the workforce included both local and non-local staff, necessitating deliberate efforts to harmonize working relationships.

Cultural Challenges
- Work-life balance conflicts
- Regional cultural practices, such as a preference for relaxed evenings, had an impact on hospital operations.
- This posed a business challenge, particularly in optimizing occupancy rates during non-peak hours.

Gap Analysis and Prioritization
- **Cost Management**: Focused on controlling redundant expenses and optimizing resource allocation.
- **Team Competencies**: A skills gap mapping exercise helped identify areas for staff development.
- **Operational Gaps**: Addressed underutilized facilities, such as the ICU and oncology departments.

Action Plan Development
- **Cost Rationalization**: Identified areas for immediate cost savings without compromising quality.

- **Revenue Optimization**: Developed marketing and patient engagement strategies to enhance visibility and retention.
- **Stakeholder Engagement**: Built relationships with government bodies and community leaders to foster mutual growth.

Strategic Interventions: Three major strategic areas were identified and addressed to enhance hospital operations:

1. Strengthening ICU Capabilities
- Upgraded training programs and equipment availability.
- Partnered with regional hospitals to improve critical care services.

2. Developing Oncology Services
- Identified a lack of modern oncology infrastructure as a strategic gap.
- Designed and implemented a business plan for comprehensive oncology services.
- Secured board approval for necessary investments.

3. Revitalizing Medical Tourism
- Redesigned marketing strategies to attract international patients.
- Focused on promoting unique hospital strengths to differentiate in a competitive market.

People-Centric Approaches

1. Hostel Facilities for Staff: Improved living conditions for nurses and medical staff to enhance morale and retention.

2. Team Building and Motivation:
- Conducted regular team meetings and collaborative activities.
- Organized celebratory events, leadership retreats, and recognition programs.

3. Performance Management:

- Transitioned from subjective to objective evaluations for fair and transparent appraisals.
- Developed middle-layer leadership to build a strong succession pipeline.

Tools and Frameworks for Execution

- **Gap Analysis Framework**: Provided a structured approach to identifying and addressing deficiencies.
- **Balanced Scorecard**: Aligned individual and departmental goals with organizational objectives.
- **SWOT Analysis**: Evaluated strengths, weaknesses, opportunities, and threats to develop actionable strategies.
- **Lean Principles**: Streamlined processes to eliminate redundancies and enhance efficiency.

Outcomes and Impact

- **Operational Efficiency:** Enhanced ICU and oncology services, positioning the hospital as a regional leader in critical care and cancer treatment.
- **Revenue Growth:** Strategic marketing and cost optimization efforts led to a significant increase in occupancy rates and improved financial performance.
- **Staff Morale**: Improved facilities and motivational programs created a more engaged workforce.

Organizational Assessment: Diagnosing Issues and Gaps

- **Departmental Misalignment**: A lack of synergy between department heads, middle management, and frontline staff hindered collaboration and efficiency.
- **External Perception Challenges**: Persistent negative media coverage and strained relationships with government agencies and local medical

professionals negatively impacted the hospital's reputation.

- **Internal Discontent**: Low morale and dissatisfaction among staff negatively affected productivity and teamwork.
- **Operational inefficiencies** arose from unclear processes and inadequate planning, resulting in financial losses and service delivery bottlenecks.

By systematically addressing these challenges through structured change management frameworks, the hospital achieved long-term sustainability, improved patient care, and enhanced organizational efficiency.

STRATEGIC TOOLS AND FRAMEWORKS FOR TURNAROUND

Team Alignment and Empowerment: A crucial aspect of the turnaround strategy was creating a cohesive and empowered team to drive transformation effectively.

1. Strengthening Leadership:
- The departmental head was positioned as a central figure in aligning teams and ensuring accountability.
- When leadership gaps were identified, corrective actions were taken, including strengthening leadership roles or replacing ineffective leaders to ensure smooth operations.

2. Support for Middle Management
- Special emphasis was placed on middle management, equipping them with the necessary tools, training, and support to implement change.
- Middle managers played a crucial role in bridging the gap between leadership and front-line employees, ensuring smooth communication and the effective execution of strategies.

3. Engaging Front-Line Employees

- Efforts were made to align front-line staff with organizational goals through monthly meetings, collaborative planning sessions, and structured feedback loops.
- These initiatives reinforced a sense of purpose, teamwork, and unity, resulting in increased efficiency and morale.

4. Succession Planning

- The development of future leaders was prioritized to ensure sustained growth beyond the current leadership's tenure.
- High-potential employees were identified and given mentorship opportunities to prepare them for leadership roles.

Fostering a Positive Ecosystem

1. Improving Staff Motivation :

- Despite delivering high-quality healthcare, the organization experienced internal dissatisfaction among its employees.
- Initiatives such as recognition programs, collaboration-building efforts, and employee engagement activities were introduced to enhance morale and workplace satisfaction.

2. Strengthening External Relationships:

- Strained relationships with local stakeholders, including government officials and referring doctors, were identified and addressed.
- Historical grievances were reviewed, and trust-building measures were implemented through proactive engagement and transparency.

3. Addressing Media Perception

- Negative media coverage was a recurring challenge that required strategic interventions.

- A focus was placed on transparent communication, showcasing positive organizational changes, and engaging with the community to enhance public perception.

Operational Efficiency
1. Cost Management
- A phased approach was implemented to optimize costs, prioritizing changes that would minimize resistance and have no adverse impact on patient care.
- Pilot programs were introduced to test cost-cutting measures, with rollback options in place in cases of significant resistance or inefficiencies.

2. Strategic Planning
- Long-term planning was incorporated into daily operations, shifting the focus beyond immediate challenges.
- The team worked on sustainable growth strategies, setting objectives for two-year expansion plans to ensure future scalability.

3. Process Improvements
- Collaborated with HR and corporate teams to enhance recruitment, training, and employee retention strategies.
- A focus was placed on building local capacity and developing workforce skills to reduce dependency on external hiring.

Navigating External Challenges
1. Government Schemes and Policy Negotiations
- A co-payment system under the DDSSY scheme was successfully negotiated with the health secretary.
- This strategic move allowed the hospital to participate in a government healthcare initiative while maintaining financial viability.

2. Expanding Market Reach
- Initiatives were launched to attract patients from neighboring states, such as Karnataka and Tamil Nadu.
- Outreach programs, referral partnerships, and targeted marketing efforts helped increase patient inflow beyond the immediate local market.

3. Stakeholder Management
- A holistic view of stakeholder interactions was adopted, recognizing that changes in one area could have a ripple effect throughout the organization.
- Special efforts were made to align stakeholders, ensuring mutual benefits and shared objectives.

Building a Resilient Culture: A culture of resilience and adaptability was instilled within the organization through consistent engagement, systematic problem-solving, and future-focused planning.

1. Field Engagement and Hands-On Leadership
- Senior management actively engaged on the ground, interacting with teams across departments.
- This hands-on approach helped identify immediate challenges, build trust, and establish rapport with employees.

2. Systematic Problem-Solving
- Challenges were addressed collaboratively, with an emphasis on team-based solutions rather than top-down directives.
- Employees were encouraged to take ownership of problems, fostering a sense of accountability and responsibility.

3. Long-Term Vision and Continuous Improvement
- A culture of continuous improvement was established, encouraging employees to seek innovation and efficiency in their daily operations.

- Future-focused planning ensured that the hospital remained adaptable to industry trends, market shifts, and evolving healthcare demands.

DIAGNOSTIC FRAMEWORKS

Identifying Gaps and Building Solutions: The initial phase of transformation required a thorough diagnostic process to identify gaps in operations, communication, and strategy. This involved extensive engagement with top leadership, middle management, and frontline staff to gain a comprehensive understanding of the hospital's challenges.

Key Findings

1. Disjointed Alignment: Poor coordination between departmental heads and frontline teams hindered operational performance and efficiency.

2. External Challenges: Stakeholder dissatisfaction and negative media narratives affected the hospital's public reputation and regulatory standing.

3. Historical Legacy Issues: Poor decisions by previous administrators created systemic challenges, including strained relationships with regulators and inefficient operational structures. These diagnostic insights underscored the need for a holistic change strategy that addressed operational inefficiencies, team dynamics, and external perceptions.

STRATEGIC PLANNING

- **Revenue and Cost Optimization**
  - **Quick Wins**: Implementing cost-saving measures that could be executed without resistance.
  - **Pilot Testing**: Introducing incremental changes on a small scale before a full-scale rollout to assess impact and feasibility.

- Evidence-Based Decision-Making: Using data-driven insights to monitor progress and make informed adjustments as needed.

A critical component of the plan involved investing in team motivation while managing costs, including improving workplace conditions and upgrading staff benefits (e.g., enhanced meal plans).

- **Long-Term Goals**
  - Expanding services to Karnataka and Maharashtra to broaden market reach.
  - Fostering a culture of continuous improvement and learning to drive operational excellence.
  - Developing future leaders who could sustain and expand the hospital's success.

LEADERSHIP AND TEAM BUILDING

- **Aligning Teams Across Levels**
  - **Empowering Department Heads**: Strengthening departmental leadership ensured better coordination with hospital-wide goals.
  - **Supporting Middle Management**: Providing resources, mentorship, and clear expectations helped bridge the gap between strategic planning and frontline execution.
  - **Engaging frontline** staff through regular team meetings, open communication forums, and recognition programs fostered a sense of inclusion, ownership, and accountability among staff.
- **Addressing External Challenges**
  - **Negative Media Coverage**: Persistent critical reports in local newspapers were tackled by enhancing service quality, engaging journalists proactively, and improving transparency.

○ **Regulatory Hurdles**: Delayed licenses and pending government scheme payments were resolved through continuous dialogue and strengthened relationships with regulatory bodies.

OUTCOMES AND LESSONS LEARNED

- **Holistic Diagnosis is Crucial**: A comprehensive understanding of financial, operational, and cultural dimensions is essential for effective decision-making.
- **Stakeholder Engagement Matters**: Building trust and collaboration with internal and external stakeholders has a profound impact on an organization's success.
- **A Framework-Driven Approach Ensures Efficiency**: Tools such as PESTEL analysis and gap analysis provide structured methodologies to identify and address key challenges.
- **Adaptability to Local Context is Key**: Understanding Kochi's unique cultural and economic dynamics, such as its reliance on tourism, was crucial for aligning services and managing the workforce.
- **Cultural Alignment Drives Organizational Effectiveness**: Adapting team-building approaches and service models to local work culture enhanced productivity and patient experience.
- **Investing in People Yields Long-Term Benefits**: Prioritizing employee well-being, development, and motivation translates into higher morale, better retention, and improved performance.
- **Strategic Foresight Ensures Sustainability**: Proactive planning helped mitigate future challenges, ensuring long-term organizational growth.
- **Continuous Improvement is Necessary for Long-Term Success**: Iterative planning, feedback mechanisms, and performance evaluations enabled sustained progress.

- **Empowered Leadership Aligns Teams Effectively**: Strong, empathetic leadership ensures team alignment, operational efficiency, and an engaged workforce.
- **Long-Term Vision Balances Immediate Challenges and Future Growth**: Sustained success requires a dual focus—addressing short-term obstacles while planning strategically for the future.
- **Collaborative Change Management Drives Sustainable Transformation**: Change was not imposed, but co-created with the team, ensuring buy-in, ownership, and reduced resistance across all organizational levels.

Through structured leadership, data-driven strategies, and a people-first approach, the hospital successfully navigated change, improved operational efficiencies, and strengthened external relationships, securing long-term sustainability and growth.

The turnaround of Alwyn Hospital in Kochi between 2016 and 2018 exemplifies the power of strategic planning, stakeholder engagement, and collaborative leadership. The hospital achieved remarkable results by diagnosing challenges, aligning teams, and building strong relationships with external stakeholders.

This case highlights the significance of a comprehensive management approach that integrates financial, operational, and cultural elements to achieve sustainable success. It serves as a guide for healthcare leaders and administrators on how to tackle complex challenges and develop resilient organizations.

WHY CHANGE MANAGEMENT IS CRITICAL IN HEALTHCARE?

Change management is essential in the healthcare sector for several critical reasons, as the healthcare environment is inherently dynamic and constantly evolving. Hospitals, clinics, and other healthcare organizations face continuous shifts due to technological advances, regulatory changes, evolving patient expectations, and economic pressures.

Here's why change management is indispensable in this sector:

- **Healthcare is a Complex and multidimensional system,** comprising multiple components, including medical technologies, patient care processes, administrative workflows, legal frameworks, and financial models. Successfully managing change in this complex environment requires careful planning and coordination to ensure all elements are aligned throughout any transformation. Without a structured change management strategy, hospitals risk compromising care delivery, patient safety, and organizational stability.

- **Adoption of New Technology and Systems**: Healthcare organizations are progressively embracing new technologies, such as electronic health records (EHRs), telemedicine, advanced medical imaging, and AI-powered tools. However, merely implementing technology is not enough. The effective integration of these innovations demands careful attention to staff training, workflow redesign, and system interoperability. Change management facilitates smooth transitions, reduces resistance, and enhances organizational adoption.

- **Regulatory and Compliance Requirements**: Healthcare is one of the most highly regulated industries worldwide. From patient data privacy (e.g., HIPAA compliance) to accreditation standards (e.g., Joint Commission), organizations must regularly update their practices to adhere to new laws, regulations, and industry standards. Change management is necessary to help healthcare organizations implement these regulatory changes without disrupting patient care or compromising compliance.

- **Evolving Patient Expectations**: Patients' expectations have undergone significant shifts in today's healthcare environment. They now demand better quality care, transparency, faster services, and more involvement in their health decisions.

  Healthcare organizations need to adapt their service delivery models to meet these expectations. Change management ensures that healthcare professionals and systems are equipped to address these evolving needs while maintaining operational efficiency and effectiveness.

CULTURAL AND BEHAVIORAL SHIFTS

Healthcare organizations are often deeply rooted in established practices and cultural norms, particularly in areas such as clinical decision-making, communication, and patient care.

Implementing any new initiative, whether a new patient care model or an organizational restructuring, often faces resistance due to ingrained behaviors and attitudes. Change management helps address this by ensuring that all stakeholders, from doctors to administrative staff, understand and accept the reasons for the change and are motivated to participate in it.

- **Staff Engagement and Morale**: Healthcare organizations rely heavily on the expertise and dedication of their staff. Without a structured change management approach, transitions may lead to staff burnout, confusion, or increased resistance. By involving staff early in the change process, providing necessary training, and maintaining consistent communication, change management fosters staff buy-in, leading to higher morale, improved performance, and better patient care.

- **Ensuring Continuity of Care**: One of the most critical aspects of healthcare is maintaining continuity of care for patients. Significant changes in medical processes, organizational structures, or technology can disrupt patient care if not managed effectively. Change management ensures that all transitions—whether upgrading systems, integrating new protocols, or reengineering workflows—are implemented without compromising patient safety or the quality of care.

- **Cost Efficiency and Resource Allocation**: Healthcare systems face increasing pressure to do more with fewer resources, necessitating cost optimization and improvements in efficiency.
  When organizations implement changes to enhance financial sustainability or operational efficiency, effective change management helps ensure that resources are allocated efficiently and potential risks are identified early, thereby minimizing waste during the transition process.

- **Facilitating Organizational Agility**: The healthcare sector is experiencing rapid shifts in market dynamics, including economic pressures, global health crises (e.g., COVID-19), and demographic changes. Healthcare organizations must be agile and capable of responding quickly to new challenges. A well-managed change process enables organizations to remain flexible and adapt to unexpected circumstances, ensuring the continued provision of quality care even in times of crisis.

- **Risk Mitigation**: Healthcare organizations face numerous risks when implementing changes, including operational disruptions, legal non-compliance, and patient safety concerns. A structured change management process ensures that risks are assessed, mitigation strategies are implemented, and all stakeholders are adequately prepared for the challenges ahead. This approach helps prevent potential legal liabilities, reputational damage, or adverse impacts on patient care.

- **Improving Patient-Centered Care**: As patient-centered care gains momentum, hospitals and healthcare providers are adopting models that emphasize individualized and holistic care approaches. Managing change is crucial for transforming an organization's culture and processes to prioritize the patient experience at all levels of care. Effective management must address resistance and actively involve staff and patients in the transformation journey to ensure these changes align with patient-first objectives.

- **Sustaining Long-Term Improvement**: Healthcare organizations face constant pressure to sustain long-term improvements. Whether upgrading the quality of care, enhancing operational performance, or achieving patient satisfaction goals, organizations must embed change into their culture and ensure it becomes an ongoing process. Through effective change management, improvements can be institutionalized and continuously refined, ultimately leading to better outcomes for both healthcare providers and patients.

Change management in healthcare is not just a beneficial strategy—it is a necessity. The healthcare sector is undergoing rapid transformations due to technological advancements, evolving regulations, and changing patient expectations. Without effective change management, these transformations will likely encounter significant barriers, including staff resistance, care disruptions, compliance failures, or financial setbacks. A well-designed change management process ensures that transitions are well-coordinated, stakeholders are aligned, and the focus remains on delivering high-quality patient care.

This structured approach is essential for healthcare organizations to adapt to change, mitigate risks, and stay competitive in an ever-evolving landscape while fostering an environment where both staff and patients thrive

4

SUSTAINABLE CHANGE MANAGEMENT

C hange is a constant in healthcare. Whether driven by advancements in medical technology, evolving regulations, or shifting patient expectations, the industry continually adapts to meet new demands.

However, despite the relentless pace of change, the nature of these transformations presents complex challenges. Healthcare change involves intricate systems, multidisciplinary teams, and established practices.

The true challenge lies in implementing these changes effectively and ensuring their long-term sustainability.

Sustainable change management goes beyond addressing immediate requirements or short-term challenges. It ensures that new processes, policies, and innovations provide lasting value while integrating seamlessly into the broader system.

THE DYNAMICS OF CHANGE IN HEALTHCARE

Healthcare is unique in its operational complexity.

Changes often stem from external pressures, such as technological advancements, policy reforms, and shifts in patient demographics.

Internally, the need for change may arise from efforts to improve efficiency, enhance patient outcomes, or address workforce challenges.

These factors make healthcare particularly susceptible to resistance and fatigue, especially when changes are frequent, poorly planned, or inadequately supported.

A defining characteristic of change in healthcare is its widespread impact on the entire system. For example, implementing electronic health records, adopting a new treatment protocol, or transitioning to value-based care often necessitates modifications across multiple departments, teams, and workflows. Consequently, effective change management requires a holistic approach. Leaders must consider the interconnectedness of various components within the system, ensuring that changes in one area do not unintentionally disrupt or weaken other parts of the organization.

DEFINING SUSTAINABLE CHANGE MANAGEMENT

Sustainable change management refers to implementing changes that address the intended challenges while remaining effective over time without excessive resource expenditure. This involves:

1. Integration with Organizational Culture: Changes should align with the organization's values and mission, fostering stakeholder acceptance and long-term commitment.

2. Scalability and Adaptability: Sustainable changes should be designed to accommodate future growth and evolve as circumstances change.

3. Stakeholder Engagement: Long-term success depends on securing the involvement and buy-in of those affected, ensuring they have the knowledge and resources to maintain the transformation.

4. Ongoing Evaluation and Support: Systems must be in place to monitor the impact of changes and address any emerging issues proactively.

PRINCIPLES OF SUSTAINABLE CHANGE MANAGEMENT

1. Vision Alignment: Every sustainable change begins with a clear vision. Leaders must clearly articulate how the change aligns with the organization's overarching goals, whether these are improving patient care, reducing costs, or enhancing staff satisfaction. This alignment helps stakeholders understand the purpose of the change and fosters a sense of shared commitment.

2. Stakeholder Engagement: Engaging stakeholders early and continuously is critical for sustainability. Healthcare organizations comprise diverse groups, including clinical staff, administrators, public health managers and patients, each with unique perspectives and concerns. Effective engagement involves:

- Communicating the "why" behind the change.
- Actively involving stakeholders in the planning and decision-making process.
- Addressing concerns and providing training to ease transitions.

For example, when implementing a new electronic health record (EHR) system, involving frontline clinicians in the selection and design process ensures the tool meets practical needs, reduces resistance, and increases adoption.

3. Resilience Building: Sustainable change requires resilience within the organization. This means creating systems and a culture that can absorb disruptions and adapt to evolving circumstances. Resilience-building strategies encompass fostering a culture of learning, encouraging innovation, and providing support to staff during challenging times.

4. Change Management Frameworks: Applying structured frameworks such as Kotter's 8-Step Change Model or Prosci's ADKAR Model provides a roadmap for navigating change.

These frameworks emphasize the importance of creating urgency, building coalitions, and reinforcing changes over time, all of which contribute to sustainability.

IMPLEMENTING SUSTAINABLE CHANGE

1. Assessing Readiness for Change: Before initiating any change, it is essential to evaluate the organization's readiness. This involves assessing factors such as organizational culture, existing capabilities, and potential barriers to success. A readiness assessment helps identify areas requiring additional support or resources.

2. Pilot Testing and Incremental Implementation: Rather than implementing large-scale changes all at once, organizations should pilot new initiatives in a controlled environment. This approach allows for testing, feedback, and adjustments before a broader rollout. Incremental implementation reduces risks and builds confidence among stakeholders.

3. Ensuring Continuous Communication: Sustained change requires continuous communication that reinforces the benefits and progress of the initiative. Communication should be transparent, frequent, and tailored to the specific needs of different stakeholder groups. Regular updates help maintain momentum and address emerging concerns.

4. Providing Training and Resources: Effective change often necessitates new skills, behaviors, and workflows. Comprehensive training programs ensure that staff can adopt and sustain changes. Additionally, ongoing support—such as access to technical assistance or peer mentoring—helps address challenges as they arise.

MEASURING AND SUSTAINING IMPACT

1. Defining Metrics of Success: Establishing clear metrics to evaluate the success of a change initiative is essential.

Metrics should be specific, measurable, achievable, relevant, and time-bound (SMART). For example, a hospital implementing a new hand hygiene protocol might track compliance rates, infection rates, and staff feedback to measure effectiveness.

2. Regular Monitoring and Feedback: Sustainability requires continuous monitoring to identify challenges and opportunities for improvement.

Feedback loops enable organizations to make data-driven adjustments, ensuring that changes remain relevant and practical over time.

3. Embedding Change into Organizational Processes: For a change to endure, it must become an integral part of the organization's routine operations. This may involve:

- Updating policies to reflect new practices.
- Integrating changes into performance evaluations and accountability structures.
- Establishing dedicated teams to oversee long-term implementation and maintenance.

4. Celebrating Success and Recognizing Contributions: Acknowledging the efforts of individuals and teams who contribute to successful change initiatives fosters a sense of accomplishment and reinforces positive behaviors. Celebrations, recognition programs, and incentives help maintain morale and commitment, ensuring long-term success.

CASE STUDY: NHS SCOTLAND CLIMATE EMERGENCY & SUSTAINABILITY STRATEGY 2022-2026

The NHS Scotland Climate Emergency & Sustainability Strategy for 2022-2026 outlines a comprehensive framework to achieve a net-zero healthcare service while addressing the climate emergency and promoting public health. The strategy focuses on five key themes: Sustainable Buildings & Land, Sustainable Travel, Sustainable Goods and Services, Sustainable Care, and Sustainable Communities. This case study examines the actions, goals, and challenges associated with implementing the strategy, as well as the broader implications for healthcare sustainability and public health in Scotland.

Objective of the Strategy: The primary goal of the NHS Scotland Climate Emergency & Sustainability Strategy 2022-2026 is to reduce the NHS's environmental impact and move towards a net-zero carbon healthcare system. The strategy outlines several ambitious actions across five main themes to ensure that NHS Scotland contributes to tackling the climate crisis while also improving the health and well-being of communities.

Key Themes of the Strategy
a. Sustainable Buildings & Land: The Sustainable Buildings & Land theme focuses on reducing greenhouse gas emissions from NHS buildings, adapting infrastructure to climate change, and ensuring responsible environmental stewardship. The strategy has set the following key objectives:
- Reduce greenhouse gas emissions from NHS buildings by at least 75% by 2030 (compared to a 1990 baseline).
- Achieve net-zero emissions for all NHS buildings by 2040 or earlier.

- Use renewable heating systems in all NHS-owned buildings by 2038.
- Improve energy efficiency and manage waste better across NHS properties.

One of the biggest challenges in achieving these goals is addressing the high energy demand of NHS buildings, which are responsible for a significant portion of the NHS's carbon emissions. The strategy calls for adapting the estate to climate impacts and managing resources more sustainably, particularly regarding green spaces, which are an asset to public health and biodiversity.

b. Sustainable Travel: The Sustainable Travel theme addresses the need to reduce the environmental impact of transportation used by NHS Scotland. Key initiatives include:

- Promoting active travel, including walking, cycling, and public transportation.
- Decarbonizing the NHS fleet, aiming to eliminate fossil-fuelled small and light commercial vehicles by 2025.

Sustainable travel reduces carbon emissions and promotes healthier communities by encouraging physical activity and improving access to healthcare services. The strategy aims to ensure that all NHS sites are accessible by public or community transport, particularly in remote and rural areas where disruption due to climate change can significantly impact service delivery.

c. Sustainable Goods and Services: This theme focuses on reducing the environmental footprint of the NHS's supply chain and promoting a circular economy. The main objectives include:

- Reducing waste through the repair, reuse, and recycling of goods and materials.
- Encouraging suppliers to reduce their greenhouse gas emissions and adopt environmentally friendly practices.
- Enhancing the resilience of the supply chain to climate change.

The NHS spends a significant amount on goods and services annually, with a large portion of its carbon footprint attributed to the manufacturing and distribution of medical equipment, chemicals, and medicines. By adopting a circular economy approach, NHS Scotland aims to mitigate these impacts by sourcing durable and recyclable products and working with suppliers to improve environmental and social sustainability.

d. Sustainable Care: The Sustainable Care theme focuses on rethinking how care is provided to make it more sustainable while improving health outcomes and reducing inequalities.

Some of the key initiatives include:

- Developing sustainable care pathways and promoting green health initiatives.
- Embracing Realistic Medicine, which focuses on delivering care tailored to the individual, promoting shared decision-making, and reducing unnecessary treatments and waste.

Reducing the environmental impact of medical practices, such as reducing emissions from inhalers, anesthetic gases, and medical waste. For example, metered-dose inhalers (MDIs) are potent greenhouse gases commonly used for asthma and chronic obstructive pulmonary disease (COPD).

NHS Scotland aims to reduce emissions from inhalers by 70% by 2028. Similarly, reducing the use of desflurane and other anesthetic gases will lower the carbon footprint of healthcare services.

d. Sustainable Communities: The Sustainable Communities theme recognizes the interconnectedness between environmental sustainability, public health, and social equity. Key focus areas include:

- Building Community Resilience to Climate Change Impacts.
- Engaging communities in sustainable practices to reduce health inequalities.
- Ensuring that health and well-being are considered in urban planning and development, including the support of green spaces and active transportation.

The strategy emphasizes that the climate emergency exacerbates existing health inequalities, particularly for marginalized and low-income communities. By collaborating with local authorities, health organizations, and other stakeholders, NHS Scotland seeks to create healthier environments and foster social sustainability.

1. Goals and Targets: The strategy outlines several ambitious goals and targets to guide NHS Scotland towards a net-zero health system:

- Net-zero greenhouse gas emissions for all NHS Scotland buildings by 2040.
- Renewable heating systems in all NHS buildings by 2038.
- Zero emissions from NHS fleets by 2030, with a complete transition to renewable-powered vehicles by 2025.
- Reduction of inhaler propellant emissions by 70% by 2028.

2. Challenges and Opportunities: While the NHS Scotland Climate Emergency & Sustainability Strategy sets clear goals, several challenges must be addressed:

- **Financial Constraints**: Implementing energy-efficient infrastructure and transitioning to renewable energy systems in NHS buildings will require significant investment. However, the long-term benefits of cost savings and improved health outcomes may offset these initial costs.
- **Behavioral Change**: Achieving the strategy's goals will require significant changes in staff and patient behavior. NHS Scotland must foster a culture of sustainability throughout the workforce and communities, ensuring that all stakeholders are aligned with the changes.
- **Rural and Remote Areas**: Climate change and infrastructure disruptions pose particular challenges for rural and remote healthcare facilities.

The strategy must ensure resilient access to healthcare services in these areas.

- **Supply Chain Management**: Encouraging suppliers to adopt sustainable practices and ensuring the availability of sustainable goods and services will require collaboration across industries and the broader public sector.

The NHS Scotland Climate Emergency & Sustainability Strategy 2022-2026 is an ambitious and comprehensive plan to address the twin challenges of the climate emergency and public health. By integrating sustainability into every aspect of healthcare delivery, from buildings and travel to the care provided and the communities served, the strategy aims to reduce NHS Scotland's environmental impact and contribute to the broader goal of a healthier, more sustainable society.

Reference: NHS Scotland. (2022). Climate Emergency & Sustainability Strategy 2022-2026.

CASE STUDY: SUSTAINING A CULTURE OF QUALITY THROUGH CHANGE MANAGEMENT IN HEALTHCARE

Healthcare organizations face constant demands to improve outcomes, enhance operational efficiency, and deliver exceptional patient care. A critical factor in meeting these demands is cultivating and maintaining a culture of quality, where quality improvement (QI) principles are embedded into organizational values, goals, and processes.

However, achieving this cultural transformation requires not only the implementation of systemic and process changes but also the effective management of human dynamics. This case study examines how a mid-sized healthcare organization transitioned to a sustainable culture of quality by implementing structured change management strategies.

By focusing on the process and human sides of change, the organization successfully navigated challenges, engaged stakeholders, and institutionalized quality as a core organizational value.

The Challenge: Building a Sustainable Culture of Quality

The healthcare organization faced several challenges that highlighted the need for a stronger quality culture:

- **Fragmented Processes**: Quality initiatives were siloed, resulting in inconsistent practices and outcomes.
- **Employee Resistance**: Staff perceived QI efforts as additional tasks, disconnected from their daily responsibilities.
- **Lack of Leadership Commitment**: While senior leaders expressed support for quality, visible engagement and accountability were limited.
- **Inadequate Training**: Employees lacked the skills and knowledge to implement and sustain QI projects.

To address these issues, the organization adopted NACCHO's Roadmap to a Culture of Quality as its guiding framework, integrating change management principles to ensure long-term success.

Phase 1: Preparing for Change - The organization began by understanding its current culture and assessing its readiness for change. This phase involved three critical steps:

- **Defining the Vision**: Leadership articulated a clear vision: to embed quality improvement into all aspects of the organization's operations. This vision emphasized that quality was not an isolated initiative but a shared responsibility aligned with patient-centered care.
- **Conducting Assessments**: Through employee surveys, SWOT analyses, and focus groups, the organization evaluated its baseline quality culture, identifying strengths such as a dedicated workforce and

weaknesses, including fragmented communication channels.

- **Identifying Change Leaders**: A multidisciplinary change management team was established, including executive leaders, managers, and frontline staff. This team served as champions for quality, driving both the strategic and operational aspects of the transition.

Phase 2: Transitioning: Transitioning involved designing and implementing specific strategies to address both process and human aspects of change.

- **Developing the Change Management Plan**: The change management team created a detailed roadmap outlining goals, timelines, and resource allocation. A comprehensive QI plan was also developed, specifying objectives such as training requirements, communication strategies, and performance metrics.
- **Communication and Resistance Management**: A robust communication plan was launched to address resistance. Early messaging emphasized creating urgency, highlighting the risks of maintaining the status quo and the benefits of adopting a culture of quality.
  - Communication channels included town hall meetings, newsletters, and targeted briefings for different employee groups. Leaders emphasized transparency and encouraged open dialogue to address concerns.
- **Training and Coaching:** Customized training programs equipped employees with QI tools and methodologies. Frontline staff were trained in practical techniques, such as root cause analysis and process mapping, while managers received coaching on leading change and fostering team buy-in.
  - Supervisors were provided with additional resources to support their teams, acknowledging their crucial role in integrating organizational strategies with day-to-day operations.

- **Implementing Process Changes**: Structural changes were introduced, including streamlining workflows and redesigning job roles to incorporate quality responsibilities.
  - A new electronic system was implemented to track QI projects and ensure department consistency and accountability.

Phase 3: Institutionalizing Change: The final phase focused on embedding quality into the organization's formal and informal culture to ensure sustainability.

- **Evaluation and Continuous Improvement**: Progress was monitored through regular audits, performance reviews, and feedback sessions. Metrics such as employee engagement, QI project success rates, and patient outcomes were tracked to assess the initiative's impact.
  - Gaps were identified and addressed through iterative adjustments, reinforcing the organization's commitment to continuous improvement.
- **Policy Integration:** Quality principles were formally integrated into policies, performance appraisals, and hiring criteria. This institutional alignment signaled that quality was a temporary focus and a foundational element of the organization's identity.
- **Celebrating Success**: Milestones and achievements were recognized through various programs, including the "Quality Champions" awards. These initiatives fostered a sense of pride and reinforced the value of quality efforts among staff.

Outcomes and Lessons Learned: Through its structured approach to change management, the healthcare organization achieved significant outcomes:

- **Improved Processes**: Adopting standardized workflows led to measurable gains in efficiency and patient outcomes.

- **Enhanced Employee Engagement**: Training and involvement in decision-making empower staff, reduce resistance, and foster a sense of ownership and accountability.
- **Leadership Commitment**: Executive leaders maintained visibility throughout the transition, modeling the behaviors they sought to instill within the organization.
- **Sustainable Quality Culture**: Quality became an integral part of the organization's strategic direction and everyday operations.

Key lessons from this case study include:
- **Balance Process and Human Factors**: Both dimensions are equally important and must be addressed concurrently for successful change to occur.
- **Engage Stakeholders Early**: Involvement fosters trust and alignment, reducing resistance.
- **Commit to Continuous Monitoring**: Regular evaluation ensures that changes remain effective and adaptable over time.

This case study illustrates that sustaining a quality culture requires a deliberate and integrated approach to change management. By addressing both the technical and human dimensions of change, the organization achieved operational improvements and laid the groundwork for ongoing excellence in patient care. Healthcare leaders can draw on these strategies to navigate their journeys toward a culture of quality, ensuring that improvements are achieved and sustained for the long term.

HEALTHCARE AND SUSTAINABLE CHANGE MANAGEMENT

Healthcare is a dynamic field where technological advances, patient needs, and regulatory requirements demand constant adaptation.

However, the success of these changes depends not just on their implementation but on their sustainability.

Sustainable change management ensures that improvements endure over time, benefiting patients, staff, and the organization as a whole. Sustainable change management is grounded in several core principles: continuity, adaptability, stakeholder engagement, evidence-based decision-making, and organizational alignment. These principles provide a foundation for creating and maintaining effective and relevant changes, even within the complexities of the healthcare environment.

Core Principles of Sustainable Change Management

1. Continuity: Continuity ensures that changes are seamlessly integrated into the organization's operations and maintained over time. In healthcare, where patient care and safety are paramount, disruptions during the implementation of change can have severe consequences.

Key Elements of Continuity:

- **Clear Vision and Goals**: Defining long-term objectives prevents mission drift.
- **Strong Leadership**: Leaders play a pivotal role in championing change and ensuring it remains a priority across departments.
- **Institutionalizing Changes**: Embedding changes into organizational policies, standard operating procedures, and performance metrics ensures long-term adoption and sustainability.

Example: A hospital implementing a new electronic health record (EHR) system aligned the rollout with existing workflows and provided extensive staff training to prevent disruptions in patient care. As a result, the new system became an integral part of operations, enhancing documentation accuracy and efficiency.

2. Adaptability: Healthcare is influenced by emerging diseases, technological innovations, and shifting patient demographics. Adaptability allows organizations to respond to these changes while maintaining the integrity of their improvements.

Key Elements of Adaptability:

- **Flexible Processes**: Designing systems that can be adjusted without losing effectiveness.
- **Feedback Mechanisms**: Regularly gathering stakeholder input to identify areas for refinement.
- **Resilience**: Cultivating a culture that embraces change and views it as an opportunity for growth.

Example: During the COVID-19 pandemic, many healthcare providers rapidly shifted to telehealth services. Organizations with adaptable systems quickly scaled up their telehealth offerings, ensuring uninterrupted patient care while maintaining high service standards.

3. Stakeholder Engagement: Achieving sustainable change requires the buy-in and active involvement of stakeholders, including healthcare providers, administrative personnel, patients, and policymakers. Engaging these stakeholders promotes ownership, minimizes resistance, and ensures that changes align with the needs of those most directly impacted.

Key Elements of Stakeholder Engagement:

- **Transparent Communication**: Keeping stakeholders informed about the change's rationale, goals, and progress.
- **Inclusive Decision-Making:** Involving representatives from all affected groups in planning and implementation.
- **Empowerment:** Providing stakeholders with the tools and authority they need to contribute effectively.

Example: A clinic seeking to improve patient appointment scheduling engaged front-desk staff and patients in redesigning the process. By incorporating their feedback, the clinic implemented a system that reduced wait times and improved patient satisfaction.

4. Evidence-Based Decision-Making: In a field as critical as healthcare, decisions must be guided by robust data and proven methods. Evidence-based decision-making ensures that changes are well-informed and more likely to achieve their intended outcomes.

Key Elements of Evidence-Based Decision-Making:
- **Data Collection and Analysis**: Using metrics to assess the current state, identify opportunities for improvement, and measure success.
- **Learning from Best Practices**: Drawing lessons from successful initiatives in other organizations.
- **Continuous Monitoring**: Evaluating the impact of changes and adjusting strategies as needed.

Example: A hospital reduced hospital-acquired infections (HAIs) by implementing a hand hygiene protocol based on evidence from research studies. Regular audits and adherence to evidence-based practices significantly decreased HAIs, enhancing patient safety.

5. Organizational Alignment: Sustainable change requires alignment between the change initiative and the organization's values, Kochils, and resources. Misalignment can lead to confusion, inefficiency, and diminished impact.

Key Elements of Organizational Alignment:
- **Strategic Integration**: Ensuring that changes support the organization's overarching mission and priorities.
- **Resource Allocation**: Providing the necessary funding, staffing, and infrastructure to sustain the change.
- **Cultural Fit**: Aligning changes with the organization's culture and fostering a mindset that supports continuous improvement.

Example: A healthcare organization focused on improving patient-centered care integrated this goal into its strategic plan. Initiatives such as staff training in empathetic communication and redesigning care processes to prioritize patient convenience, aligned with the organization's mission, reinforced the desired cultural shift.

Application of the Principles in a Healthcare Setting

- **Improved Patient Outcomes**: Sustainable change reduces errors, enhances care quality, and fosters better health outcomes.
- **Operational Efficiency**: Integrated and well-maintained changes streamline workflows, saving time and resources.
- **Staff Satisfaction and Retention**: Engaged and empowered employees are more likely to support and sustain improvements.
- **Organizational Resilience**: Flexible and adaptive systems enable organizations to respond effectively to future challenges.

Scenario: Implementing a Patient Safety Initiative

An extensive hospital network sought to enhance patient safety through a system-wide initiative aimed at reducing medication errors. Applying the principles of sustainable change management, the organization:

- Ensured continuity by integrating the initiative into its strategic goals and policies.
- Built adaptability by designing protocols that could be modified as new evidence emerged.
- Engaged stakeholders in developing and testing solutions, including nurses, pharmacists, and patients.
- Used evidence-based decision-making to identify high-risk areas and measure the effectiveness of interventions.
- Achieved organizational alignment by prioritizing patient safety in resource allocation and staff training.

The Result: A significant reduction in medication errors, increased staff confidence, and enhanced patient trust.

Creating Lasting Change in Healthcare: Focusing on continuity, adaptability, stakeholder engagement, evidence-based decision-making, and alignment allows healthcare organizations to create lasting change.

These principles drive improvements and build a foundation for progress. Sustainable change management ensures initiatives remain relevant, helping organizations navigate a complex landscape while delivering high-quality care. By embedding these principles, leaders can turn challenges into opportunities for excellence.

SUSTAINABLE CHANGE MANAGEMENT IN HEALTHCARE – INSIGHTS FROM COL M RAJGOPAL

Sustainable change management is essential for the healthcare sector, where continuous improvement and adaptability are paramount. Col M Rajgopal emphasized the importance of institutionalizing cultural values, leveraging existing structures, and striking a balance between urgency and long-term planning.

This case study encapsulates these insights, offering actionable strategies for healthcare leaders to navigate the complexities of change management effectively.

The Challenge: Moving Beyond Individual Leadership: Col M Rajgopal began by emphasizing the need to shift the focus from personality-driven leadership to institutional frameworks. While visionary leaders can drive significant progress, over-reliance on individual charisma risks derailing efforts when leadership changes. He remarked,

"Cultural values must be institutionalized, not tethered to individuals. A leader's departure shouldn't mean the end of a good initiative."

Key Insights

1. Sustainability Over Personality: For long-term success, organizations must embed cultural values into their DNA. Leadership transitions should not disrupt progress.

Sustainable change involves creating policies, workflows, and performance metrics that perpetuate desired behaviors, irrespective of who leads the organization.

2. Leveraging Legacy Structures: Existing systems and influential stakeholders can act as catalysts for change. Instead of dismantling legacy structures, Col M Rajgopal advocated working within them and adapting processes to align with new objectives.

3. Balancing Crises and Gradual Change: While crises can act as a springboard for rapid change by providing a sense of urgency, they often lack the staying power of carefully planned initiatives. Col M Rajgopal stressed the importance of deliberate, proactive change:

"A crisis might ignite the flame, but sustained change is a slow burn—built steadily, brick by brick."

Drawing from his extensive experience, Col M Rajgopal outlined five actionable strategies to achieve sustainable change in healthcare organizations:

1. Integrate Leadership Development: Leadership development should begin early, embedding training into healthcare management education. Future leaders must strike a balance between clinical expertise and managerial acumen to navigate complex systems effectively.

2. Elevate HR's Role: Human Resources (HR) should evolve into a strategic partner, actively driving change initiatives. From workforce planning to fostering a culture of accountability, HR plays a pivotal role in sustaining progress.

3. Foster Advocacy: Senior leaders must champion change initiatives, serving as visible role models. Their advocacy can galvanize organizational buy-in, making change more palatable to employees.

4. Encourage Public-Private Collaboration: Knowledge-sharing between the public and private sectors is vital. Public systems can adopt innovative practices from the private sector, while private entities benefit from the public sector's broader reach and policy influence.

5. Focus on Longevity: Systems and processes should be designed to adapt over time, ensuring continuity even in the face of leadership or stakeholder turnover. This involves establishing a robust foundation of institutional knowledge and cultivating organizational resilience.

To illustrate these principles, Col M Rajgopal shared a case from his tenure in hospital management. A central healthcare facility faced declining service quality due to inconsistent leadership and fragmented processes. By applying the recommendations outlined above, the organization transformed its culture and operations:

- **Leadership Development**: A leadership training program was introduced, targeting mid-level managers. This program emphasized a blend of clinical and managerial skills, preparing participants for future leadership roles.

- **HR Transformation**: HR was restructured to include strategic planning capabilities. This shift empowered the department to play a proactive role in change management and employee engagement.

- **Advocacy**: Senior leaders, including Col M Rajgopal, actively participated in communication campaigns, town halls, and training sessions to champion the change process.

- **Public-Private Collaboration**: The hospital partnered with private sector consultants to implement new patient care workflows, leveraging best practices to enhance efficiency.

- **Sustainability Measures**: Policies and performance metrics were revised to ensure alignment with the new vision. Succession planning was prioritized to prevent leadership gaps.

Within two years, the facility achieved significant improvements in patient satisfaction, employee engagement, and operational efficiency. This case study underscores the importance of institutionalizing values, leveraging legacy systems, and maintaining a balanced approach to change. Key takeaways include:

- Leadership should not only initiate change but also build mechanisms to sustain it.
- Legacy structures can be assets when appropriately aligned with new goals.
- Sustainable change is incremental, requiring persistence and strategic foresight to achieve lasting results.

Col M Rajgopal reveals that sustainable change management in healthcare hinges on a blend of visionary leadership, robust systems, and a long-term perspective. By adopting these principles, organizations can navigate the complexities of the healthcare sector, achieving not just transformation but enduring success.

POLICY TO ACTION CASE STUDY: COMMUNITY HEALTH OFFICERS (CHOS) IN INDIA BASED ON A DISCUSSION WITH DR SHWETA SINGH

This case study examines the evolution and implementation of the Community Health Officer (CHO) program under India's Comprehensive Primary Health Care (CPHC) initiative, a cornerstone of the Ayushman Bharat scheme. Drawing on an in-depth conversation with **Dr Shweta Singh**, a key technical expert who worked closely with both national and state-level institutions, the study offers first hand insights into how a nationally driven policy was transformed into action on the ground.

From policy formulation to training roll-out and state-level adoption, Dr Shweta's reflections reveal the complex interplay of political will, institutional coordination, and frontline realities that shaped the success and challenges of the CHO initiative.

To expand access to comprehensive primary healthcare in rural and underserved areas by deploying **mid-level healthcare providers (MLHPs)** known as **Community Health Officers (CHOs)** at Health and Wellness Centres (HWCs) under the **Ayushman Bharat** scheme.

1. **Policy Background**
   - The **National Health Policy 2017** emphasized **Comprehensive Primary Health Care (CPHC)**.
   - CHO was conceptualized as the **mid-level provider** to deliver 12 packages of essential services at HWCs.
   - Rooted in earlier models from **Chhattisgarh (RMA)** and **Assam (RHP),** where local candidates were trained to serve in remote areas.

2. **Policy Design and Development**
   - A formal committee under the Ministry of Health designed the CHO program.
   - Collaboration with IGNOU for curriculum development.
   - Two committees created: one each for **nursing graduates** and **Ayurveda graduates**.
   - **Key national documents** guiding implementation:
     - Task Force Report on CPHC
     - CPHC Implementation Framework

3. **Cultural and Structural Challenges**
   - **State's response varied**:
     - Some (like southern states in India) had financial and technical independence. Others were hesitant due to a lack of capacity, fear of fund underutilization, and pressure to meet targets.

- Initial **uncertainty and confusion** about how to implement CHO selection, training, and integration.
- **Indira Gandhi National Open University (IGNOU) slow administrative process** delayed roll-out by nearly a year.

4. **Stakeholder Landscape**
   - **National Stakeholders:**
     - Ministry of Health and Family Welfare (MoHFW)
     - IGNOU (education partner)
     - NHSRC (technical agency)
   - **State-Level Stakeholders:**
     - State Health Department
     - State NHM Mission Directors
     - State training institutions
   - **Enablers:**
     - Strong, stable leadership from national officers
     - Political mandate tied to the launch of Ayushman Bharat.
     - Full **financial support through NHM** (dedicated budget head).
     - Continuous **handholding from the NHSRC**, with state consultants assigned to guide roll-out.

5. **Implementation Pathway**
   - NHSRC and MoHFW developed and shared:
     - Prototypes of advertisements for candidate recruitment
     - Screening/eligibility criteria
     - Training and monitoring templates
   - CHOs were recruited, trained, and deployed across states.
   - Emphasis on **local recruitment** to enhance retention and community trust.

6. **Key Enablers of Success**
   - **Political will**: Strong push from the central government to implement and scale up.
   - **Dedicated leadership**: Long-standing senior officials provided continuity.
   - **Incentives to states**: Financial incentives to encourage states to adopt.
   - **Integration into NHM**: Ensured long-term sustainability and funding.

7. **Challenges and Adaptations**
   - Delays due to **bureaucratic hurdles** with IGNOU and state approvals.
   - States initially resisted due to fear of penalties for unspent funds.
   - Variation in state capacity led to uneven adoption and quality of services.
   - Lack of early focus on **quality assurance** and **career progression** for CHOs.
   - **Implementation was rushed due to the ambitious 1.5 lakh HWC target, leading** to "on-paper" compliance in some areas.

8. **Monitoring and Evaluation**
   - Early monitoring relied on field visits, phone check-ins, and review meetings.
   - Monthly updates tracked:
     - Candidate enrolment
     - Budget spending
     - Program center functionality
   - Recently, digital monitoring tools and NQAS standards have been introduced.

9. **Sustainability Measures**
   - Structural integration: HWCs and CHOs are now part of the national health infrastructure.
   - Community expectations: As services expand, reversal

becomes politically infeasible.

- Ongoing discussions on:
  - ○ Expanding CHO prescribing rights
  - ○ Building CHO career pathways

10. Lessons Learned
- **What Worked Well:**
  - ○ Centralized leadership and coordination
  - ○ Financial backing through the NHS
  - ○ Identification of motivated "champions" at the state level
  - ○ Use of existing models (Chhattisgarh, Assam) as an evidence base.

What Could Improve:
- More phased, quality-focused implementation
- Clearer CHO career progression paths
- Earlier development of monitoring frameworks
- Stronger focus on **equity and motivation** of CHOs, many of whom are on contract

The CHO initiative marks a landmark shift in India's primary healthcare landscape, transitioning from **facility-centric care** to **community-based, preventive services**. While the program faced bureaucratic and implementation hurdles, it succeeded primarily due to **political commitment**, **stable leadership**, and **robust inter-agency coordination**. Continued focus on **quality, motivation, and sustainability** will be critical to its long-term impact.

EMBEDDING CHANGE INTO ORGANIZATIONAL CULTURE

Sustainable change management in healthcare is not a one-time effort or a series of isolated projects; instead, it requires integration into the very fabric of an organization's culture.

Organizational culture refers to the shared values, beliefs, and behaviors that guide decision-making and actions.

For change to have a lasting impact, it must become part of this culture. In healthcare, where patient care, safety, and service quality are critical, embedding change into the culture is essential for ensuring long-term success.

To make change sustainable, it must be deeply integrated into the organization's daily operations, values, and norms.

This involves engaging key stakeholders, aligning the change with the organization's mission and values, and ensuring leadership consistently supports and models the new behaviors. Only through these actions can change be institutionalized in a way that endures, becoming a driving force for continuous improvement.

How to Embed Change into Organizational Culture

Embedding change into a healthcare organization's culture involves several strategic actions. These actions help align new behaviors and practices with the organization's core mission, ensuring that the change is not temporary or dependent on a specific leader but becomes an enduring aspect of the institution.

1. Aligning Change with Organizational Values: For change to be effectively embedded, it must align with the organization's existing values and mission. This alignment makes the change feel like a natural extension of the organization's purpose, ensuring buy-in from employees at all levels. Leaders must communicate how the change supports the organization's vision and goals. When change is consistent with the organization's values, employees are more likely to adopt it.

Example: If a healthcare organization's mission emphasizes patient-centered care, a change initiative that aims to improve patient communication through better technology would align with that value. The change becomes part of the organizational DNA, reinforcing the commitment to patient care.

2. Engaging Stakeholders: Effective stakeholder engagement is crucial for embedding change into the organization's culture. Stakeholders include senior leadership, frontline staff, patients, and external partners. Change should not be imposed top-down without input; instead, it should be a collaborative process that involves stakeholders in decision-making, planning, and implementation. When employees have a say in the changes that affect their work, they are more likely to take ownership of the initiative and integrate it into their daily routines.

Key Engagement Strategies:

- **Transparent Communication**: Provide clear, consistent messaging about the change.
- **Regular Meetings**: Facilitate discussions between leadership and staff to promote open communication and collaboration.
- **Feedback Loops**: Provide multiple channels for employees to express their concerns.
- **Open Forums**: Create spaces where employees can discuss challenges and offer suggestions for improvements.

Example: A hospital introducing a new patient scheduling system actively sought input from nurses, administrative staff, and patients. By incorporating their feedback, the hospital developed a system that was both user-friendly and efficient, resulting in higher adoption rates and reduced resistance.

3. Training and Development: For change to become part of the organizational culture, employees must be equipped with the necessary skills and knowledge to adopt new practices. Training and development are key to making change a part of everyday behavior.

Key Aspects of Training:

Comprehensive Education Programs: Help employees understand why the change is happening.

- **Hands-On Training**: Ensure staff can practically apply new skills.
- **Ongoing Support**: Provide mentorship, refresher courses, and troubleshooting resources.

Example: A hospital adopting a new electronic health records (EHR) system provided extensive training programs for physicians, nurses, and administrative staff. This ensured that staff could use the system efficiently, integrating it into daily healthcare workflows.

4. Leadership Commitment and Modeling: Leadership plays a pivotal role in embedding change into the organizational culture. Leaders must not only support the change but also model the desired behaviors.

Key Leadership Strategies:

- **Lead by Example**: Leaders should actively participate in the change process.
- **Communicate the Vision**: Provide a clear roadmap for transformation.
- **Recognize Achievements**: Celebrate milestones and progress.
- **Offer Continuous Support:** Address employee concerns promptly and effectively.

Example: A hospital's executive leadership team actively participated in EHR training sessions alongside frontline staff. Their visible commitment to learning the new system reinforced its importance, ensuring that employees embraced the change rather than resisted it.

5. Reinforcement Through Policies and Systems: To make change a permanent part of the culture, it must be reinforced through organizational systems and policies. This includes embedding the new practices into performance appraisals, incentive structures, and everyday workflows. For example, if the change focuses on patient safety, the organization might revise its policies to prioritize safety in staff evaluations and performance reviews.

Regular audits, feedback mechanisms, and performance monitoring are essential for maintaining accountability. Recognizing and rewarding behaviors that align with the change ensures that the new practices remain valued within the organization.

Benefits of Embedding Change into Organizational Culture

1. **Consistency**: When change is deeply integrated into the culture, it becomes consistent across the organization. All employees, from leadership to frontline staff, work toward the same goals, ensuring uniformity in patient care and organizational performance.

2. **Resilience**: A culture that embraces change is more adaptable to future challenges. Healthcare organizations that embed change management practices are better equipped to respond to unforeseen crises, regulatory changes, or technological advancements.

3. **Continuous Improvement**: When change is institutionalized, it fosters an environment of continuous improvement. Staff members are more likely to identify areas for further development and innovation, which drives ongoing progress and keeps the organization ahead of industry trends.

4. **Enhanced Employee Engagement**: Embedding change into the culture gives employees a sense of ownership in the process. They feel more involved and invested in the organization's success, which leads to higher morale, job satisfaction, and retention rates.

5. **Improved Patient Outcomes**: Ultimately, when change is embedded in the culture, it results in better care delivery. Healthcare providers are more likely to follow best practices, leading to improved patient safety, satisfaction, and overall health outcomes.

Embedding change into the organizational culture is critical for ensuring that change initiatives have a lasting impact. By aligning changes with organizational values, engaging stakeholders, providing training, and ensuring leadership commitment, healthcare organizations can create a culture that adapts to change and thrives on it.

CASE STUDY: UNDERSTANDING THE DYNAMICS OF SUSTAINABLE CHANGE – A 20-YEAR CASE STUDY OF INTEGRATED HEALTH AND SOCIAL CARE

Change management is a significant challenge in healthcare, particularly in areas where integration of services is required, such as health and social care. One of the most critical areas of change within healthcare systems involves integrating health and social care services for people with complex needs, such as those with mental health issues. Achieving sustainable integration in these areas is challenging, as many initiatives struggle to maintain their effectiveness over the long term. Integrated health and social care involves coordinating healthcare services with social support systems to provide holistic care to individuals, particularly those with multifaceted needs. This integration is crucial to improving patient outcomes, reducing redundancies, and ensuring continuous care. However, sustainable integration remains elusive in many healthcare systems due to the complexities of managing change across different organizational structures and sectors. Previous research has primarily focused on the initial stages of integration, such as the initiation, resistance, and implementation phases. At the same time, longitudinal studies that track the sustainability of these changes are limited. This case study examines a 20-year initiative focused on integrated health and social care. The study focuses on a model organization operated under national policy directives. It illustrates the dynamics that contributed to sustainable change in service delivery for people with complex mental health and social care needs.

Study Objectives: The study's objective was to explore the dynamics behind sustainable change in the integration of health and social care. Specifically, it aimed to understand the actions and processes that contributed to the long-term sustainability of the integration efforts. The study was grounded in the Dynamic Sustainability Framework (DSF), a tool that enables an in-depth examination of the factors influencing the sustainability of organizational changes.

Methodology

A qualitative case-study design was employed, with data collected through analyzing the steering committee minutes from the model organization. The data spanned a period from 1995 to 2015, providing a comprehensive view of the evolution of integration efforts and the key factors that supported their long-term sustainability. The Dynamic Sustainability Framework (DSF) was used as a conceptual lens for analyzing the data. The DSF is a comprehensive approach that considers the interplay of various factors, such as organizational structure, leadership, resources, and stakeholder engagement, that contribute to the sustainability of change initiatives.

Findings

The study revealed that the key to long-term sustainability in integrated health and social care was the development of inter-sectoral cooperation. This was achieved through a participatory approach, where various stakeholders, including service users, healthcare providers, and social care organizations, collaborated to design and refine the service model. Key findings include:

1. **Shared Structure for Cooperation:** A shared structure was created to facilitate cooperation between health and social care services.
2. This structure supported continuous quality improvement and learning, ensuring that services were aligned with the evolving needs of the service users.

It became apparent that ongoing learning, based on real-time feedback, was crucial to maintaining the effectiveness of the integration efforts.

3. **Cooperation Across Organizational Levels:** One of the key principles of the integration effort was cooperation at all organizational levels.

   This included cooperation between different organizational units within the healthcare and social care sectors, as well as the involvement of service users, stakeholder associations, and other partner organizations. This collaborative culture helped establish a foundation for sustainability, as all involved parties were invested in the change process.

4. **Service User Involvement:** A major contributor to sustainable integration was the consistent and active involvement of service users in the decision-making process. Service user involvement ensured the services were tailored to their specific needs, leading to higher satisfaction and better outcomes. Regular reviews of service users' needs allowed the organization to adapt its approach as required, ensuring that services remained relevant and practical over time.

5. **Contextual Adaptation of Change Content:** Another critical finding was the need for continuous refinement of the content to suit the context in which it was being implemented. The study demonstrated that continuously adapting and evolving the integration efforts was more effective than designing a fixed change model at the pre-implementation stage. This flexibility allowed the organization to respond to emerging challenges and opportunities, ensuring that the integration process remained dynamic and relevant to the needs of the population served.

Implications for Practice

The findings from this case study have several important implications for healthcare managers and policymakers seeking to implement and sustain integrated health and social care models, especially for individuals with complex mental health and social care needs.

1. **Emphasizing Participatory Approaches**: It is crucial to involve all stakeholders, especially service users, from the outset of any integration initiative. This ensures that the services meet the real needs of the target population and encourages stakeholder buy-in, which is essential for long-term success. The participatory approach also fosters a sense of ownership among all parties involved, which is crucial for overcoming resistance and ensuring sustainability.

2. **Ongoing Quality Improvement and Learning**: Building a structure that supports continuous learning and quality improvement is essential for sustaining change. Integrating health and social care must be viewed as an ongoing process, where regular feedback from service users and frontline staff informs adjustments and improvements. This helps the organization adapt to changing needs and challenges, ensuring the system remains effective over time.

3. **Adaptability and Flexibility**: The ability to adapt to changing circumstances and needs is critical for the sustainability of integrated care. Rather than committing to a rigid, one-size-fits-all model, healthcare organizations should focus on refining and adapting their integration strategies as they go. This means being open to new ideas, processes, and technologies to enhance care delivery and improve outcomes.

4. **Cross-Sector Cooperation**: Effective integration of health and social care requires cooperation not only within each sector but also across sectors.

Healthcare and social care organizations must collaborate to create a seamless care experience for individuals with complex needs.

This requires shared goals, joint planning, and a commitment to ongoing communication and collaboration. This case study provides valuable insights into the dynamics of sustainable change in integrated health and social care. Through a participatory approach, service user involvement, and ongoing adaptation to contextual needs, the organization maintained and refined its integration efforts over 20 years.

These efforts were guided by the principles of cooperation, continuous improvement, and responsiveness to change, which are essential for creating a dynamic and sustainable care system. The study highlights that while integrating health and social care is challenging, it is possible to achieve long-term sustainability by focusing on adaptability, stakeholder engagement, and a commitment to continuous learning.

References: Klinga, C., Hasson, H., Andreen Sachs, M., & Hansson, J. (2020). Understanding the dynamics of sustainable change: A 20-year case study of integrated health and social care. Journal of Health Management, 65(3), 321-337.

CASE STUDY: TRANSFORMING CARE SYSTEMS IN THE CONTEXT OF THE SUSTAINABLE DEVELOPMENT GOALS (SDGS) AND OUR COMMON AGENDA

Care is fundamental to the well-being, prosperity, and sustainability of individuals, societies, economies, and ecosystems. It encompasses a broad spectrum of activities, from providing care to individuals within households to more formalized healthcare systems that support entire populations. The importance of care becomes clear when considering that every individual requires care at different stages of their life.

Effective care systems ensure that individuals of all ages and their diverse needs can participate fully in society, access services that fulfill their needs, and exercise their rights. Moreover, the care system is not limited to personal or healthcare needs; it also extends to caring for the environment, which is integral to the sustainability of life on Earth. A sustainable care system requires balancing human needs with environmental considerations, ensuring that the quality of life of current generations does not compromise that of future ones. However, despite its essential role, care work often goes undervalued, particularly in terms of its economic and social worth, which limits investment and policy focus. This case study explores the challenges and opportunities associated with transforming care systems, as outlined in the United Nations system policy paper on the SDGs and Our Common Agenda. It highlights the inequities in care systems, with a particular focus on gender disparities, the impact of the COVID-19 pandemic, and the role of care in achieving the Sustainable Development Goals (SDGs).

The Gendered Divide in Care Work

Globally, care work is disproportionately carried out by women and girls. More than 75% of unpaid care work is performed by women, with women spending an average of 4 hours and 25 minutes per day on care tasks, compared to 1 hour and 23 minutes for men. The gendered division of care work is rooted in deeply entrenched social norms and gender stereotypes, which frame women as the primary caregivers in the household and men as the primary breadwinners. This division extends into both unpaid and paid care work, resulting in disparities in the recognition and compensation of care work.

The undervaluation of care work is further compounded by the economic model, which often overlooks unpaid care work in national accounts, such as GDP, despite its significant contribution to economies. The unpaid care work performed by women and girls is estimated to contribute between 2% and

41% of a country's GDP, with a median value of 10%. On a global scale, this amounts to an estimated $10.8 trillion annually.

However, despite its immense value, care work, especially unpaid, rarely receives adequate policy attention or financial investment.

COVID-19 Pandemic: The Fragility and Inequality of Care Systems

The COVID-19 pandemic underscored the vital role that care workers—especially women—play in sustaining the functioning of society. During the pandemic, care continued, even as much of the global economy came to a halt. The pandemic disproportionately affected women, who were more likely than men to reduce their paid work hours or exit the workforce entirely due to increased care responsibilities at home. In 2020, school and preschool closures added 672 billion hours of additional unpaid childcare globally, with women shouldering 76% of those hours.

At the same time, the pandemic exposed the fragile and unequal nature of existing care systems. For example, people with disabilities and older adults, particularly those in institutional settings, were disproportionately affected by the health crisis. However, despite the increased reliance on unpaid and underpaid care work, only 7% of the social protection and labor market measures implemented during the pandemic supported unpaid care work. This highlights the need for large-scale investments in comprehensive care systems to ensure resilience in future crises.

The Need for Comprehensive Care Systems

As global demographics change, the demand for care services is growing. The number of people aged 65 and older is expected to double by 2050, with significant challenges facing low- and middle-income countries. At the same time, there is a growing demand for childcare services, with approximately 350 million children worldwide needing access to childcare. These trends underscore the pressing need to transform and invest in comprehensive care systems that are sustainable, equitable, and capable of meeting the diverse needs of various populations.

Transforming care systems is not simply about increasing funding for healthcare services, but about reimagining how care is provided, valued, and how it can contribute to broader societal goals, including achieving the United Nations' Sustainable Development Goals (SDGs). The SDGs, particularly Goals 5 (Gender Equality) and 3 (Good Health and Well-being), emphasize the importance of equitable access to quality care for all individuals and the need to acknowledge and address the gendered aspects of care work.

Who Provides Care?

Women and girls are the primary providers of unpaid and paid care work globally. The gendered nature of care work is particularly pronounced in countries with limited public services, basic infrastructure, or social protection systems. In such settings, unpaid care work often falls primarily on women, especially in rural areas or single-parent households. This inequity restricts women's opportunities for education, decent paid work, public life, and leisure, creating a cycle of poverty and financial dependency.

In the paid care sector, women represent two-thirds of the workforce, including workers in healthcare, childcare, disability care, and domestic work. Many of these workers are migrants, and their labor is often undervalued and poorly compensated. Care jobs are often viewed as "unskilled" or an extension of women's "natural" caregiving roles, which contributes to their low status and pay. This undervaluation of care work has significant consequences for the workers and the recipients of care. For example, in sub-Saharan Africa, over 900,000 community health workers support the healthcare system, with the majority being women and many working without pay.

Addressing the Care Crisis: Transformative Solutions

- **Investing in Care Infrastructure**: Governments must prioritize investment in paid and unpaid care systems. This includes increasing funding for healthcare services, expanding access to childcare, and providing social protection measures for care workers. Expanding access to affordable and quality care is crucial for reducing the burden on women and improving overall societal well-being.

- **Revaluing Care Work**: A significant transformation is needed to reframe the value of care work in economic and social terms. This means recognizing the contribution of unpaid care work in national economic accounts, improving working conditions for care workers, and addressing the gendered divide in care responsibilities.

- **Empowering Women and Girls**: To break the cycle of gendered inequality in care, it is essential to promote women's participation in the workforce, provide access to education, and ensure that women have control over their time and resources. This can be achieved by promoting equal sharing of care responsibilities, expanding access to affordable care services, and ensuring that men are equally involved in caregiving.

- **Building Resilient Care Systems:** The COVID-19 pandemic demonstrated the fragility of care systems and the vulnerability of care workers, especially women. Governments and international organizations must collaborate to develop more resilient healthcare systems that can withstand future crises. This includes ensuring adequate support for informal care workers, increasing investment in the care sector, and strengthening social protection mechanisms to support them.

Transforming healthcare systems is crucial for achieving the Sustainable Development Goals (SDGs) and building a more just and sustainable world. It requires addressing the deeply embedded gender inequalities in care work, investing in comprehensive and resilient care systems, and revaluing the essential work of caregivers.

The need for equitable and sustainable care systems will only increase as the world continues to face demographic shifts and global challenges, such as pandemics and climate change.

Through coordinated action, governments, international organizations, and civil society can establish care systems that support individuals and societies while upholding human rights and promoting sustainable development.

References: United Nations (2021). Transforming Care Systems in the Context of the Sustainable Development Goals and Our Common Agenda. UN System Policy Paper.

ENSURING LONG-TERM SUCCESS THROUGH MONITORING AND SUSTAINABILITY

Implementing change within an organization, particularly in complex fields like healthcare, is just the first step toward improvement. To ensure that the change is not only practical but also sustainable over time, it is crucial to monitor progress continuously and make necessary adjustments. Monitoring and evaluating the impact of change initiatives allow organizations to assess the success of the changes and determine if they are achieving the desired outcomes. Additionally, sustainability requires ongoing efforts to maintain the momentum of change, ensuring that it continues to benefit the organization and its stakeholders.

The Importance of Monitoring and Evaluation

After a change initiative is launched, the organization must closely track its effects to confirm its effectiveness and that it is achieving its intended objectives. Monitoring and evaluation are essential as they enable the early detection of potential issues, assess the success of changes against their goals, and identify areas that require modification. Without proper monitoring, an organization may remain unaware of the change's success or where improvements are needed.

Monitoring and evaluation can be accomplished through various methods, including:

- **Regular Audits** – Periodic audits allow organizations to review performance against established standards and benchmarks. In healthcare, this could involve evaluating patient satisfaction, service quality, or operational efficiency.
- **Feedback Loops** – Collecting input from staff, patients, and stakeholders is crucial for evaluating the impact of changes. This feedback can be gathered via surveys, focus groups, or interviews and is vital for identifying areas that need additional attention.
- **Performance Metrics** – Using key performance indicators (KPIs) provides measurable data on specific outcomes, such as reductions in patient wait times, improvements in care quality, or financial sustainability.

These tools help organizations stay on track and make data-driven decisions to fine-tune the changes they have introduced.

The Ongoing Efforts Required to Sustain Change

Sustaining change is not a one-time effort; it requires ongoing initiatives to maintain the improvements that have been achieved. Simply implementing a change is insufficient if the organization does not actively integrate it into daily operations. Sustaining change requires continuous support and commitment from leadership, as well as active participation from employees at all levels.

Key Strategies for Sustaining Change

- **Ongoing Training and Education** – After implementing changes, it is essential to conduct regular training sessions to maintain staff's skills and confidence in their new roles.

For instance, when introducing a new healthcare technology or system, providing continuous professional development opportunities ensures employees remain informed about best practices, new features, and troubleshooting methods.

- **Regularly Revising Objectives** – To ensure that the changes align with the organization's evolving needs, it is crucial to review objectives periodically. This process enables the organization to assess the ongoing relevance of its initial goals, identify emerging challenges, and explore new opportunities for improvement.

- **Engagement and Reinforcement** – One of the most critical aspects of sustaining change is maintaining high levels of engagement and morale. Leadership must consistently reinforce the benefits of the change and recognize the efforts of those involved in the transition. Celebrating small wins and making staff feel valued ensures ongoing buy-in and commitment.

For example, a healthcare organization that introduced a patient-centered care model may hold quarterly workshops or roundtable discussions to gather insights from healthcare providers and patients. This approach keeps the focus on patient care, reinforces the importance of the change, and ensures that the model adapts to patients' evolving needs.

Creating a Culture of Continuous Improvement

To fully integrate change into an organization's culture, the mindset must shift from viewing "change as a one-time event" to seeing "change as an ongoing process." Fostering a culture of continuous improvement ensures that monitoring and sustaining change become essential components of the organization's operations. In a hospital environment, a culture of continuous improvement may involve:

- **Regular Performance Reviews** – Conducting annual or semi-annual performance reviews to assess progress on key change initiatives. These reviews should include evaluating specific goals, identifying challenges, and assessing the effectiveness of solutions implemented.

- **Knowledge Sharing** – Encouraging employees to share their experiences and lessons learned from implementing change. This can be achieved through internal newsletters, meetings, or knowledge-sharing platforms where best practices are shared and exchanged.

- **Adaptation and Flexibility** – Change initiatives must be flexible enough to accommodate feedback and evolving needs. Organizations can ensure that changes align with both short-term goals and long-term strategic vision by remaining adaptable.

CASE STUDY: MAKING CHANGE LAST: APPLYING THE NHS INSTITUTE FOR INNOVATION AND IMPROVEMENT SUSTAINABILITY MODEL TO HEALTHCARE IMPROVEMENT

In healthcare, achieving sustainable change is an ongoing challenge. Although evidence-based treatments and innovative practices are essential for providing high-quality care, especially as populations age and healthcare demands increase, embedding these practices into routine care remains difficult. Variability in outcomes, often due to inconsistent implementation, is a common issue in healthcare systems worldwide. To address this, the NHS Institute for Innovation and Improvement developed the Sustainability Model (SM) to guide healthcare teams in identifying key determinants of sustainability and implementing new practices into everyday care routines. This case study examines the application of the SM within the National Institute for Health Research Collaboration for Leadership in Applied

Health Research and Care for Northwest London (CLAHRC NWL), with a focus on understanding how the model was implemented, the challenges faced, and the lessons learned for sustaining healthcare improvements over time.

Background: Implementing evidence-based treatments is crucial for aging populations and addressing the increasing healthcare demands, particularly in areas such as chronic disease management. However, applying these treatments across healthcare systems is often hindered by challenges such as resource constraints, staff turnover, and resistance to change. For improvements to be truly effective, they must become part of the organizational culture and practice. The NHS Institute's Sustainability Model (SM) was designed to address these challenges. It provides a structured approach for healthcare teams to consider the factors influencing the sustainability of healthcare improvements. The model aims to help teams recognize barriers to sustainability and take concrete actions to embed changes into their routine practice, ensuring they are sustained.

The NHS Institute's Sustainability Model
- **Leadership Commitment**: The extent to which leadership is invested in and supports the change.
- **Organizational Culture**: Whether the organization is open to change and innovation, and is aligned with values that support long-term improvement.
- **Capacity and Resources**: The availability of time, staff, and financial resources to support change.
- **Stakeholder Engagement**: Involvement of all relevant stakeholders (e.g., staff, patients, and the community) in the change process.
- **Feedback and Monitoring:** Mechanisms to measure and evaluate progress and make necessary adjustments based on data.

- **Systems and Processes**: Whether the new practices are integrated into existing workflows and systems.

The Application of the Sustainability Model in Northwest London

The **CLAHRC NWL** initiative aimed to apply the SM to various healthcare improvement projects across Northwest London. The goal was to test the model's effectiveness in encouraging sustainable change and to determine how well teams could apply its principles in practice. The evaluation involved collecting data from 19 project teams that used the SM to assess and guide their change processes. The team's engagement with the model was assessed based on their responses to the SM framework and formal progress reviews. Each team was classified into one of three categories:

- **Engaged**: Teams that consistently applied the SM to drive sustainability and made significant progress embedding changes.
- **Partially Engaged**: Teams that used the SM intermittently made some progress but lacked consistent implementation.
- **Non-Engaged**: Teams that made little to no use of the SM in their change processes.

Findings: Engagement and Challenges

Of the 19 teams that participated, the results indicated varying levels of engagement with the model. The teams were categorized as follows:

- Six teams were classified as 'engaged,' meaning they used the model consistently and made significant progress in embedding changes into routine practice.
- Six teams were categorized as 'partially engaged,' indicating that they applied the model sporadically, leading to some progress but not a consistent application.

- Seven teams were labeled as 'non-engaged,' meaning they did not use the SM consistently, and their progress in embedding sustainable practices was limited.

The study also revealed that 12 out of the 19 teams found the SM acceptable to some extent, suggesting that while the model was helpful in theory, its practical application was challenging for many teams.

Reasons for Variation in Engagement

- **Understanding and Application**: Some teams struggled to fully understand and apply the model effectively in their specific healthcare contexts. This was particularly true for teams with limited experience in using structured frameworks for sustainability.
- **Perceived Usefulness:** Feedback from certain team members suggested that they did not immediately see the benefits of using the model, resulting in sporadic use and a lack of motivation to continue using it consistently.
- **Resource Constraints**: Some teams faced challenges due to limited resources—both in terms of time and personnel—which hindered their ability to fully engage with the model and implement its recommendations.
- **Leadership and Commitment**: Teams with strong leadership support and a commitment to change were more likely to successfully apply the model. In contrast, teams without clear leadership support struggled to gain traction and faced difficulties embedding changes.
- **Diversity of Opinion:** The teams' varied opinions on the utility of the SM also contributed to differences in engagement.

The diversity of opinions gradually reduced over time, indicating that teams began to develop a more unified understanding of the model's usefulness as they applied it.

Key Lessons Learned and Recommendations

While the SM provided a valuable framework for promoting sustainable healthcare improvements, the findings highlighted several key lessons:

- **Capacity Building:** Teams required more support in capacity building and facilitation. Those with access to facilitation and training on the model's application were more likely to succeed in embedding changes.
- **Tailoring the Model**: Some teams found the structure challenging to apply directly to their unique healthcare settings. Tailoring the model to meet the specific needs and contexts of different teams and healthcare environments could improve engagement and effectiveness.
- **Leadership and Engagement**: Strong leadership and clear commitment to change were essential for success. Healthcare organizations must ensure that leaders are actively involved in guiding and supporting the implementation of sustainability efforts.
- **Continuous Feedback and Adjustment:** Regular monitoring and feedback are crucial for sustaining change. Teams need continuous data to assess progress and identify areas where additional support is needed.
- **Training and Education**: Ongoing training and education on sustainability principles, the SM, and its application are necessary to help teams effectively implement the model. This training should be tailored to the team's level of experience and the specific healthcare challenges they face.

Applying the NHS Institute for Innovation and Improvement Sustainability Model within CLAHRC NWL provides valuable insights into the challenges and opportunities of sustaining healthcare improvements. The findings suggest that while the SM has potential, its successful application depends on factors such as leadership commitment, capacity building, and tailored support for teams.

For sustainability models to be truly effective, they must be flexible, accessible, and adaptable to the needs of individual healthcare settings. Continuous evaluation, ongoing support, and a focus on capacity building are essential for ensuring that healthcare improvements are implemented and sustained over time.

References: Doyle, C., Howe, C., Woodcock, T., Myron, R., Phekoo, K., McNicholas, C., Saffer, J., & Bell, D. (Year). Making change last: Applying the NHS Institute for Innovation and Improvement Sustainability Model to healthcare improvement.

CASE STUDY: SUSTAINABILITY OF PUBLIC HEALTH INTERVENTIONS – IDENTIFYING GAPS AND ADDRESSING CHALLENGES

Background: Public health interventions are designed to address pressing health issues at the population level, but ensuring their long-term sustainability remains a complex challenge. These interventions often require significant investments in terms of resources, community involvement, and policy support. While many interventions may show initial success, the ability to maintain their impact over time is a critical aspect that can determine their overall effectiveness.

The research by Walugembe, Sibbald, Le Ber, and Kothari (2020) explores the concept of sustainability in public health interventions, addressing the gaps in understanding and strategies that hinder the long-term success of these initiatives.

This case study examines the issues presented in their research, highlighting the challenges and potential solutions to enhance the sustainability of public health programs.

The Need for Sustainable Public Health Interventions

Public health interventions aim to improve the overall health of populations, reduce health disparities, and address significant health issues, including chronic diseases, infectious outbreaks, and mental health crises. However, the effectiveness of an intervention is not solely measured by its short-term success but by its ability to create lasting change.

Sustainability in public health refers to the continued effectiveness and maintenance of an intervention long after the initial implementation phase. The challenge of sustainability is not merely about keeping interventions running but ensuring that they continue to provide value over time. Several factors contribute to the challenge of sustaining public health interventions, including limited financial resources, shifting political landscapes, changes in community priorities, and difficulties in maintaining stakeholder engagement.

Key Challenges Identified in Walugembe et al. (2020)

Walugembe and colleagues (2020) identify several critical gaps and challenges that hinder the sustainability of public health interventions. These challenges include variations in how sustainability is conceptualized, the lack of standardized frameworks for measuring sustainability, methodological difficulties, and challenges in reporting and evaluating sustainability.

Variations in Conceptualizing Sustainability: One of the primary challenges in sustaining public health interventions is the lack of a universally accepted definition of sustainability. Different stakeholders—researchers, policymakers, funders, and community members—may have varying interpretations of what sustainability means in practice.

This variability in definitions complicates efforts to measure and evaluate sustainability across different public health initiatives.

Sustainability can encompass a range of elements, such as:

- **Program outcomes**: The extent to which health improvements continue to be observed after the initial intervention.
- **Community engagement**: The ongoing involvement of the community in maintaining and supporting the intervention.
- **System integration**: The degree to which the intervention becomes integrated into local health systems or broader public health policies.

Without a shared understanding of what sustainability entails, it becomes challenging to design interventions that can achieve a lasting impact.

Lack of Standardized Measurement Frameworks: Another significant gap in sustaining public health interventions is the absence of standardized frameworks for assessing sustainability. Walugembe et al. (2020) emphasize that sustainability is a multidimensional concept that necessitates a nuanced approach to measurement and evaluation. However, most public health interventions lack agreed-upon metrics or indicators to track their sustainability over time.

Some models, such as **the Dynamic Sustainability Framework** (DSF), aim to address these gaps by providing a more flexible and context-specific approach to sustainability. However, these frameworks are not universally adopted, and there remains no consensus on the most effective methods for measuring sustainability across diverse public health contexts.

- **Methodological Challenges:** Studying the sustainability of public health interventions poses significant methodological challenges. These include issues related to longitudinal data collection, the complexity of evaluating long-term outcomes, and the difficulty in isolating the effects of interventions from other external factors that may influence health outcomes. These challenges make it difficult to track whether an intervention has maintained its effectiveness over time and whether it has adapted to the evolving needs of the community.

- **Reporting and Timing Issues.** The timing of sustainability assessments is another challenge. Sustainability is a long-term process, and it is difficult to assess the ongoing impact of an intervention without sufficient follow-up. Additionally, the reporting of sustainability outcomes is often inconsistent across studies, making it challenging to compare findings and identify best practices. Some interventions may report on short-term successes without adequately addressing long-term sustainability.

- **Proposed Solutions and Recommendations.** To address the identified challenges, Walugembe et al. (2020) propose a series of recommendations to enhance the sustainability of public health interventions. These recommendations emphasize the use of theoretically informed approaches, refining measurement frameworks, and enhancing stakeholder engagement.

- **Theoretically Informed Approaches.** One of the key recommendations for improving sustainability is the use of theoretically informed approaches in the design, implementation, and evaluation of public health interventions. Walugembe and colleagues emphasize the importance of frameworks such as the Normalization Process Theory (NPT) and the Dynamic Sustainability Framework (DSF), which provide structured approaches for understanding how interventions can be effectively embedded into healthcare systems and communities for long-term impact.

- **Normalization Process Theory** (NPT) focuses on integrating interventions into everyday practices. Sustainability is more likely when interventions become normalized and embedded into the routine processes of health systems or communities. NPT emphasizes four key components: coherence (understanding the goals), cognitive participation (engagement from stakeholders), collective action (resource support), and reflexive monitoring (ongoing evaluation).

- **The Dynamic Sustainability Framework** (DSF), on the other hand, acknowledges the evolving nature of sustainability. It recognizes that interventions must adapt to changing circumstances, such as shifts in the political or economic landscape, and remain relevant to community needs.

- **Developing Clear Metrics for Sustainability Walugembe et al.** (2020) recommend the development of clear, standardized metrics for assessing sustainability. By establishing agreed-upon criteria, such as the continued effectiveness of health outcomes, stakeholder engagement, and the integration of interventions into health systems, it will be easier to measure the success of sustainability efforts. These metrics should be flexible enough to account for the unique contexts of different public health programs but standardized to allow for comparisons across studies.

Strengthening Community Ownership and Engagement

A significant factor in the long-term success of public health interventions is the level of community ownership. Interventions that are designed in collaboration with local communities and that build local capacity are more likely to be sustained. Walugembe et al. (2020) emphasize the importance of fostering community engagement at every stage of the intervention process, including design, implementation, and evaluation.

Community ownership ensures that there is local investment in the intervention's success, thereby increasing the likelihood of continued support and resources.

Improving Cross-Sector Collaboration. Public health interventions often span multiple sectors, including healthcare, education, and social services. To improve sustainability, there needs to be better coordination and collaboration across these sectors. Walugembe et al. (2020) highlight the need for a more integrated approach, where public health initiatives are supported by both governmental and non-governmental organizations, healthcare providers, and community groups. These collaborations help secure additional resources, provide ongoing support, and ensure that interventions remain relevant to changing needs.

CASE STUDY: EMRI 108 – A SUSTAINABLE PUBLIC-PRIVATE PARTNERSHIP MODEL FOR EMERGENCY MEDICAL SERVICES IN INDIA

Background: Emergency Management and Research Institute (EMRI), launched in 2005 in Andhra Pradesh, India, represents one of the most successful examples of a sustainable public-private partnership (PPP) in healthcare. Operating under the brand "108 Emergency Service," EMRI provides integrated emergency response for medical, police, and fire emergencies across multiple Indian states. The initiative exemplifies how strategic change management and cross-sector collaboration can deliver scalable, high-impact, and sustainable public health outcomes.

The Change Vision: At inception, emergency medical services (EMS) in India were fragmented and underdeveloped. The EMRI initiative aimed to establish a standardized, accessible, and affordable emergency response system.

This vision was grounded in principles of equity, efficiency, and sustainability, aligning with broader goals of improving public health and increasing access.

Key Elements of Sustainable Change

1. Public-Private Partnership Model: EMRI's model combines public sector funding with private sector innovation and operational execution. While state governments fund the operations, EMRI, initially supported by the Satyam Foundation and later by the GVK Foundation, manages the technology, logistics, and training, ensuring agility and efficiency.

2. Scalability and Adaptability: The program began in one state but rapidly scaled across India, covering over 20 states and union territories. Each implementation was tailored to local needs while preserving core service standards. This modular and adaptable approach ensured relevance across varied socio-geographic contexts.

3. Technology Integration: EMRI introduced GPS-enabled ambulances, centralized call centers, and standardized triage protocols. These innovations enabled real-time coordination, improving response times and facilitating more effective resource utilization, which is crucial for sustainability and trust.

4. Workforce Development and Training: A strong focus was placed on paramedic training, soft skills, and continuous learning, ensuring frontline readiness and quality service delivery. This investment in human resources helped embed the change culturally and operationally.

5. Evidence-Based Monitoring and Evaluation: EMRI consistently used data analytics to monitor call volume, response time, and patient outcomes. These metrics informed both continuous improvement and evidence-based policymaking by partner governments.

6. Community Engagement and Equity: Services were provided free of cost, including in underserved and rural areas. Through awareness campaigns, EMRI gained community trust and participation, key to long-term utilization and support.

Outcomes and Impact
- Over 750 million people have access to 108 services across India.
- EMRI has responded to more than 200 million emergencies and helped save over 2.3 million lives (as reported in its impact assessments).

The initiative has become a replicable model for other countries exploring public-private partnerships (PPPs) in healthcare.

Sustainability Insights
- EMRI's success illustrates how sustainable change in healthcare hinges on:
- Clear vision and strategic alignment.
- Adaptive partnerships with shared accountability.
- Institutionalization through training, governance, and technology.
- Consistent stakeholder engagement, from policymakers to patients.

By embedding change through systems thinking, resource alignment, and continuous innovation, EMRI transformed India's emergency response landscape, proving that sustainable change is achievable at scale, even in resource-constrained settings.

References
- GVK EMRI Official Reports (www.emri.in)
- Lahariya, C. (2012). 'Strengthening Emergency Medical Services in India: Lessons from EMRI'. Indian Journal of Public Health.

- NITI Aayog. (2018). Public-Private Partnership for the Health Sector.
- Rao, K. D., & Pilot, E. (2014). 'Health systems in India: Opportunities and challenges for innovations'. Journal of Health Organization and Management.

Sustainable change management integrates changes into an organization's core for lasting effects. By emphasizing sustainability, healthcare organizations boost efficiency, enhance patient care, and improve staff satisfaction while lowering their environmental impact. This approach ensures lasting improvements that contribute to resilience and success. Effective and sustainable change requires strategic planning, stakeholder involvement, and ongoing monitoring. By aligning organizational objectives with sustainable practices, such as reducing carbon emissions and optimizing resource utilization, companies establish a strong foundation for sustainable growth. These initiatives enable organizations to proactively address external challenges, such as climate change, while enhancing their internal adaptability and resource efficiency.

The long-term benefits are substantial. Organizations that prioritize sustainability achieve cost savings through improved energy efficiency, reduced waste, and enhanced supply chain management. They also enhance their reputation as leaders in corporate social responsibility, attracting patients, employees, and partners who value sustainability. Most importantly, sustainable systems enhance public health by reducing environmental harm and promoting community well-being.

Sustainable change management is vital for healthcare organizations to thrive now and remain relevant in the future. Embracing sustainability fosters resilience, innovation, and the ability to address complex and evolving challenges.

5

APPLYING LEADERSHIP AND CHANGE MANAGEMENT IN THE TRANSFORMATION OF HEALTHCARE SETTINGS

The rapidly evolving healthcare landscape presents both unique opportunities and challenges. Technological advancements, demographic shifts, evolving disease trends, and economic pressures necessitate significant changes in the delivery of healthcare. However, the success of these changes hinges on a crucial factor: customizing initiatives to fit the specific context of different healthcare environments and settings.

THE SPECTRUM OF HEALTHCARE SETTINGS

Healthcare settings are diverse and multifaceted, encompassing institutions and organizations that vary in size, purpose, and operational complexity. These settings range from large tertiary Brooks Hospitals and specialized clinics to small community health centers, medical colleges, and public health organizations. Each operates within its unique set of constraints, goals, and challenges:

- **Hospitals**: Large, complex institutions with hierarchical structures. They manage acute and chronic illnesses, characterized by high patient volumes, fast-paced decision-making, and a strong focus on clinical outcomes.
- **Clinics**: Smaller than hospitals, clinics offer specialized or general medical care with an emphasis on efficiency and patient-centered service, often with fewer administrative layers.
- **Medical Colleges and Teaching Hospitals**: These institutions strike a balance between patient care, education, and research, creating unique challenges in aligning academic priorities with clinical needs.
- **Public Health Organizations**: Focused on population health rather than individual patient care, these entities engage in preventive care, policy advocacy, and community outreach, necessitating broad collaboration across multiple sectors.

THE NEED FOR CONTEXT-SPECIFIC TRANSFORMATION

Healthcare transformation is a complex and highly dependent process, heavily influenced by the specific environment in which changes are implemented. Each healthcare setting possesses unique characteristics that necessitate customized approaches:

- **Organizational Culture**: The internal culture of a large hospital differs significantly from that of a small clinic. Understanding these cultural differences is key to fostering engagement and reducing resistance to change.
- **Resource Availability**: Resources vary significantly between institutions. A tertiary hospital may have access to cutting-edge diagnostic equipment and specialist personnel, whereas a rural clinic may struggle with limited staff and out dated infrastructure.

Adapting transformation strategies to match available resources ensures practicality and feasibility.

- **Stakeholder Priorities**: Patients, healthcare providers, and administrators often have differing priorities, depending on their specific healthcare setting. Effective change management must account for these diverse priorities, ensuring alignment, collaboration, and consensus-building to achieve successful outcomes.

LEADERSHIP IN HEALTHCARE TRANSFORMATION

Effective leadership is at the core of any successful healthcare transformation. Leaders serve as visionaries, strategists, and motivators, guiding their organizations through complex changes. Key leadership principles essential for healthcare transformation include:

- **Visionary Leadership**: Leaders must articulate a clear and compelling vision for transformation. This vision should resonate with stakeholders at all levels and align them toward common goals.
- **Adaptive Leadership**: Given the dynamic nature of healthcare, leaders must be flexible, responding to evolving circumstances with agility and resilience.
- **Collaborative Leadership**: Healthcare transformation often involves multiple departments and disciplines. Collaborative leadership fosters teamwork and integration, breaking down silos that hinder progress.
- **Transformational Leadership**: This leadership style inspires and empowers teams to exceed expectations. Transformational leaders cultivate a culture of innovation and continuous improvement.

CASE STUDY: CHANGE MANAGEMENT IN MEDICAL INSTITUTIONS - AN IMPLEMENTATION VIEW

Change in medical institutions is a process that involves reshaping attitudes, values, and behaviors among staff to adapt to new methods and systems. As outlined by Said Elshama in his article, "Change Management in Medical Institutions: Implementation View," leading change in medical schools and healthcare systems demands effective leadership capable of navigating complex conditions. This case study builds upon Elshama's insights, providing an illustrative scenario to demonstrate practical applications of change management principles.

Background: In a prominent medical school within a large healthcare institution, a decision was made to transition from traditional lecture-based teaching to a problem-based learning (PBL) curriculum. This decision aimed to enhance student engagement and prepare graduates for the complexities of modern healthcare. However, the institution faced significant resistance from faculty accustomed to traditional methods.

Challenges Identified: The implementation of PBL in this medical school encountered several challenges:

- **Resistance to Change**: Faculty members expressed concerns about the efficacy of PBL, doubted their ability to adapt, and feared additional workload.
- **Organizational Culture**: The institution favored established hierarchies and conventional teaching methods, creating barriers to innovation.
- **Resource Constraints**: The limited availability of trained facilitators and financial resources complicated the transition process.
- **Stakeholder Misalignment**: Some students and staff members were skeptical about the benefits of PBL, resulting in a lack of enthusiasm for the approach.

Strategic Approach: Drawing from Elshama's framework, the institution adopted a structured change management strategy to address these challenges:

- **Urgency and Vision**: The leadership team articulated a compelling vision for the change, emphasizing the need to align medical education with global best practices. They highlighted the gap between current outcomes and desired future states, creating a sense of urgency among stakeholders.
- **Stakeholder Engagement**: A core team was formed, including faculty champions, student representatives, and administrative staff. This team facilitated open dialogues, allowing stakeholders to voice concerns and contribute ideas, fostering a sense of ownership.
- **Capacity Building**: Faculty development workshops were organized to train educators in PBL methodologies. External experts were invited to share success stories and provide technical assistance.
- **Short-Term Wins**: Pilot programs were initiated in select departments. These pilots demonstrated tangible benefits, including improved student performance and satisfaction, which encouraged the broader adoption of this approach.
- **Institutional Alignment**: Policies and resources were realigned to support the PBL approach.

Overcoming Resistance: Resistance to change was addressed through multiple strategies:

- **Transparent Communication**: Regular updates were provided to all stakeholders, addressing misconceptions and showcasing progress.
- **Incentives**: Faculty members who excelled in PBL facilitation were recognized and rewarded, motivating others to participate.
- **Support Systems**: A mentoring program paired

experienced faculty with those new to PBL, providing guidance and reassurance.

Results Achieved: Within three years, the institution successfully transitioned to a problem-based learning (PBL) curriculum. Key outcomes included:

- **Improved Engagement**: Student participation in learning activities increased significantly.
- **Enhanced Faculty Skills**: Faculty members reported improved teaching competencies and job satisfaction.
- **Positive Reputation**: The institution's innovative approach attracted talented students and faculty, enhancing its standing in the academic community.

Lessons Learned: The case study highlights critical factors for successful change management in medical institutions:

- **Leadership Commitment**: Strong and consistent leadership is vital for driving change.
- **Tailored Strategies**: Approaches must align with the institution's unique culture and context.
- **Continuous Evaluation**: Regular feedback and adjustments ensure the change process remains on track.
- **Stakeholder Collaboration**: Inclusive planning and implementation foster trust and cooperation, promoting a more effective and efficient approach.

This case study demonstrates that effective change management can transform medical institutions despite resistance and resource constraints. Leaders can achieve sustainable improvements in education and healthcare delivery by applying structured frameworks and prioritizing stakeholder engagement.

Reference: Elshama SS. Change Management in Medical Institutions: Implementation View. Iberoam J Med. 2021;3(2):161-168. doi:10.5281/zenodo.4610269.

UNDERSTANDING THE SPECIFIC NEEDS OF DIFFERENT HEALTHCARE SETTINGS

Healthcare transformation is a multifaceted endeavor that requires a nuanced understanding of the environments in which changes are implemented. Each healthcare setting is distinct, with unique characteristics that influence patient care, operational efficiency, and organizational outcomes. Before undertaking transformation strategies, it is imperative to grasp these specific needs and challenges to design effective and sustainable interventions.

The Unique Characteristics of Healthcare Settings: Healthcare settings encompass a broad spectrum of institutions, each tailored to serve diverse populations and address varied medical needs. Key characteristics include:

1. Patient Demographics: Urban hospitals serve diverse populations with varied medical conditions, while rural clinics cater to smaller, more homogenous populations that often face resource shortages and accessibility issues. **For example**, Pediatric hospitals focus on young patients with specialized needs, requiring child-friendly facilities and expertise in pediatric care.

2. Operational Structures: Large hospitals operate with hierarchical systems and multiple departments, requiring coordination across varied specialties. In contrast, standalone clinics often have flat organizational structures with streamlined operations.

For example, Medical colleges and teaching hospitals integrate patient care, education, and research, balancing academic priorities with clinical responsibilities.

3. Regulatory Requirements: Public health organizations follow broader population health mandates, while private practices prioritize individual patient care within specific legal and insurance frameworks.

Compliance varies based on location and type of care provided, making it essential for organizations to align transformation efforts with relevant regulatory frameworks. Understanding these nuances ensures that transformation strategies are tailored to fit each setting's mission, resources, and challenges.

Why Context Matters: Transformation efforts that overlook the specific context of a healthcare setting risk failure due to misalignment with organizational realities. Contextual understanding is critical for several reasons:

- **Stakeholder Engagement**: Tailored approaches foster trust and buy-in from staff, patients, and administrators.
- **Resource Optimization**: Recognizing resource constraints allows for pragmatic planning and prioritization.
- **Regulatory Adherence**: Ensuring compliance with local and national regulations prevents legal and operational setbacks.

For example, a strategy designed for a high-tech urban hospital may not be feasible or practical in a resource-limited rural clinic. Without considering these differences, well-intentioned reforms can lead to inefficiencies, staff resistance, and poor patient outcomes.

LEADERSHIP AND CHANGE MANAGEMENT PRACTICES IN HEALTHCARE TRANSFORMATION

Healthcare systems worldwide face unprecedented challenges and opportunities in the modern era. The pressure for transformation within these systems is immense, driven by technological advancements and demographic shifts. This transformation relies on the application of effective leadership and change management practices.

These practices are not merely supportive tools; they are integral to achieving sustainable improvements in healthcare outcomes.

CASE STUDY: OVERCOMING CHANGE AVERSION IN ORGANIZATIONAL TRANSFORMATION

Organizational change is inevitable in the context of institutional growth and adaptation, but it is often met with employee resistance or aversion. Jason A. Hubbart's research highlights the challenges associated with change aversion—a psychological and behavioral response to organizational change—and provides valuable insights into mitigating these challenges to foster successful change initiatives.

This case study examines a real-world scenario inspired by Hubbart's findings, emphasizing strategies to address change aversion and enhance organizational adaptability.

Background: The ABC Medical Center, a mid-sized hospital with approximately 500 employees, faced declining patient satisfaction scores and increasing operational costs. Leadership identified outdated administrative workflows and inefficient patient care processes as key contributors to these issues.

The proposed solution involved a comprehensive transformation initiative, including the implementation of electronic health records (EHR), restructuring of care delivery models, and updates to staff training programs.

While the leadership team was confident in the benefits of these changes, they encountered significant resistance from employees across departments.

Change aversion manifested as:
- **Fear of the Unknown**: Many employees were unfamiliar with EHR systems and worried about their ability to adapt to them.

- **Loss of Control**: Nurses and administrative staff expressed concerns about losing autonomy in their workflow.
- **Preference for Familiarity**: Senior employees were particularly resistant, preferring traditional paper-based systems.

Understanding Change Aversion

Hubbart (2023) defines change aversion as an instinctive reaction to avoid organizational change due to fear of the unknown, discomfort, or cognitive rigidity. In ABC Medical Center's case, these factors were evident in employees' responses, particularly among those with long tenures who viewed the changes as disruptive rather than beneficial. Understanding these reactions required the leadership to recognize underlying psychological barriers, such as:

- **Routine Seeking**: Employees accustomed to established workflows resisted changes that disrupted their routines.
- **Emotional Reactions**: Frustration and anxiety about new technologies and processes heightened resistance.
- **Cognitive Rigidity**: Employees struggled to perceive the potential long-term benefits of the proposed changes.
- **Short-Term Focus**: Immediate discomfort overshadowed the long-term benefits of improving patient care and reducing costs.

Leadership Response: Effective leadership was critical in addressing change aversion at ABC Medical Center. Drawing on strategies identified by Hubbart and other organizational change theorists, the leadership team implemented a multifaceted approach:

i. Communicating the Vision:

- Leadership organized town hall meetings and department-specific workshops to articulate the need for change. They emphasized the gap between the current state of operations and desired outcomes, such as improved patient satisfaction and streamlined workflows.

- By framing the changes as essential to maintaining the hospital's competitive edge and service quality, they helped employees see the bigger picture.

ii. Building Trust and Empathy

- Managers conducted one-on-one meetings with employees to understand their concerns and provide reassurance. These conversations fostered trust and demonstrated the organization's commitment to supporting staff during the transition.
- Senior leaders shared their learning experiences with new technologies, modeling a willingness to embrace change.

iii. Providing Training and Support

- Comprehensive training sessions were tailored to employees' roles, ensuring they felt confident using the new EHR system.
- On-site technical support teams were available during the initial implementation phase to address issues promptly and reduce frustration.

iv. Creating a Culture of Inclusion

- Employees were invited to participate in decision-making processes, such as customizing Electronic Health Record (EHR) workflows to meet departmental needs.
- By involving staff in planning and implementation, leadership reduced feelings of imposition and increased buy-in.

v. Celebrating Early Wins

- Short-term milestones were established to demonstrate progress, such as reduced patient wait times and improved data accuracy.

- Success stories were shared through internal newsletters and staff meetings, reinforcing the value of the changes.

Outcomes: Over six months, ABC Medical Center observed significant progress:

- **Increased Employee Buy-In**: Post-implementation surveys revealed that 85% of employees felt more comfortable with the EHR system and recognized its benefits.
- **Improved Patient Satisfaction**: Patient feedback scores improved by 20%, with many citing smoother administrative processes and more personalized care.
- **Operational Efficiency Gains**: The hospital reported a 15% reduction in administrative costs and a 10% increase in care delivery efficiency.

These outcomes validated the leadership's approach to addressing change aversion and underscored the importance of strategic planning and empathetic leadership in organizational transformation.

Discussion: The case of ABC Medical Center illustrates key principles for overcoming change aversion:

- **Proactive Leadership**: Early engagement with employees to address fears and concerns can prevent resistance from escalating into entrenched opposition.
- **Tailored Solutions**: Training and support must be customized to meet the diverse needs of employees, ensuring they feel equipped to navigate the changes effectively.
- **Fostering Inclusivity**: Involving employees in decision-making empowers them to take ownership of the change process, reducing feelings of imposition.
- **Emphasizing Benefits**: Highlighting short-term successes and long-term advantages helps employees shift their focus from discomfort to opportunity.

These principles align with Hubbart's assertion that understanding and addressing the root causes of change aversion can lead to cultural acceptance and positive organizational outcomes. By prioritizing empathy, communication, and collaboration, leaders can turn resistance into a catalyst for growth.

Organizational change is inherently challenging, but it also presents opportunities for growth and innovation. The experience of ABC Medical Center demonstrates that with thoughtful leadership and strategic planning, even deeply ingrained change aversion can be overcome. As Hubbart (2023) emphasizes, fostering a culture of acceptance and adaptability is essential for navigating the complexities of modern organizational environments. Organizations can successfully transform and thrive in an ever-evolving landscape by addressing resistance with empathy, providing robust support, and celebrating progress.

Reference: Hubbart, J. A. (2023). Organizational Change: The Challenge of Change Aversion. Administration Sciences, 13(162). https://doi.org/10.3390/admsci13070162

Understanding Transformation in Healthcare Settings

Transformation in healthcare refers to significant changes aimed at improving patient care, operational efficiency, and organizational sustainability. These changes may involve adopting new technologies, restructuring workflows, or implementing policy reforms. However, transformation efforts often face resistance due to the complex and dynamic nature of healthcare environments. Each healthcare setting—hospitals, primary care clinics, public health organizations, long-term care facilities, and academic medical centers—has its unique operational structure, patient demographics, and regulatory requirements. Effective transformation requires tailored approaches that take these nuances into account.

For instance, a large urban hospital may focus on integrating advanced diagnostic tools and electronic health records (EHRs), while a rural clinic may prioritize improving access to care through telemedicine. Similarly, public health organizations may concentrate on addressing population health challenges, such as managing infectious disease outbreaks or implementing vaccination campaigns. Understanding the specific needs and challenges of each setting is the foundation for successful transformation.

The Role of Leadership in Healthcare Transformation

Leadership is the driving force behind successful healthcare transformation. Leaders set the vision, inspire teams, and create an environment conducive to change. In healthcare, leadership involves navigating complex stakeholder landscapes, balancing clinical and operational priorities, and fostering a culture of innovation and collaboration.

- **Vision and Strategic Direction**: Healthcare leaders must clearly articulate a vision for transformation that aligns with the organization's mission and addresses key challenges. For instance, a hospital CEO might aim to reduce patient readmission rates by 20% over five years, utilizing initiatives such as care coordination and data analytics.

- **Building Trust and Collaboration**: Successful leaders build trust with stakeholders, including providers, administrators, patients, and policymakers. Cooperation is essential in multidisciplinary settings where teams work together to achieve goals. For example, a chief medical officer (CMO) might engage clinicians in a quality improvement project through clear communication and inclusive decisions.

- **Emotional Intelligence and Resilience**: Healthcare leaders need to demonstrate emotional intelligence and resilience. They must manage conflict, address resistance to change, and support morale during uncertainty, especially among overwhelmed frontline staff.

- **Change Management Principles in Healthcare**: Change management offers a framework for implementing and sustaining transformation. It helps guide individuals, teams, and organizations through change to ensure adaptations are embedded in the culture.

- **Assessing Readiness for Change**: Before initiating transformation, healthcare organizations should assess their readiness by evaluating the culture, staff attitudes, and available resources. For instance, an assessment may show clinicians support adopting an EHR system but lack the required training and infrastructure.

- **Stakeholder Engagement**: Engaging stakeholders is key to effective change management. Early involvement can alleviate concerns, build support, and reduce resistance. Methods like focus groups and surveys encourage engagement. For example, including nurses and administrative staff in the reorganization of patient intake processes can lead to more widely accepted solutions.

- **Communication Strategies**: Consistent and transparent communication is vital during times of change. Leaders should clearly explain the rationale for transformation, outline the benefits, and provide regular updates. Effective communication also involves listening to feedback. In public health campaigns, clear messaging about vaccinations can help counter skepticism.

- **Training and Capacity Building**: Training and capacity-building initiatives equip healthcare professionals with the necessary skills and knowledge to deliver effective healthcare services. For new clinical protocols, hospitals might offer workshops, simulations, and coaching to ensure compliance.

- **Monitoring and Evaluation**: Ongoing monitoring and evaluation are crucial for measuring the impact of transformation and identifying areas for improvement. Key performance indicators, such as patient satisfaction and infection rates, provide valuable insights. Feedback loops allow data-driven adjustments to sustain progress.

CHALLENGES AND STRATEGIES FOR SUCCESS

- **Resistance to Change:** Resistance is a common barrier to healthcare transformation, often stemming from fear of the unknown, a loss of control, or skepticism about the benefits. Leaders can mitigate this by fostering trust, involving stakeholders in decision-making processes, and demonstrating tangible results, also known as 'quick wins'.
- **Resource Constraints:** Healthcare organizations frequently face financial and resource limitations. Creative problem-solving and strategic prioritization are vital. Leveraging public-private partnerships or applying for grants can enhance funding for transformation initiatives.
- **Balancing Short-Term and Long-Term Goals:** Leaders must strike a balance between immediate results and long-term sustainability. Short-term achievements, like reducing wait times or improving staff satisfaction, can build momentum for larger efforts.
- **Addressing Resistance**: Resistance is a natural response to significant transformation initiatives. In healthcare, the challenge is heightened by the sector's complexity, the critical nature of its services, and the diverse range of stakeholders. Effectively addressing this requires a strategic approach involving leadership, stakeholder engagement, and adaptive change management techniques.

Transformation in healthcare is complex and requires effective leadership and change management. By understanding the needs of various healthcare settings, engaging stakeholders, and using structured frameworks, organizations can overcome challenges and achieve sustainable improvements. Leaders who inspire trust, promote collaboration, and emphasize continuous learning can drive meaningful transformation and deliver high-quality care in a changing landscape.

UNDERSTANDING RESISTANCE IN HEALTHCARE

Resistance to change often stems from psychological, cultural, and systemic factors. In healthcare, unique challenges may include:

- **Disruption of Established Workflows**: Clinicians and staff may fear that new processes or technologies will interfere with their ability to deliver care efficiently.
- **Fear of the Unknown**: Healthcare professionals often prefer tried-and-tested methods, and uncertainty can create anxiety.
- **Lack of Trust**: Historical failures in implementing changes can lead to skepticism among employees.
- **Diverse Stakeholder Needs**: Physicians, nurses, administrative staff, and patients may have conflicting priorities and needs.
- **High-Stakes Environment**: Any perceived risk to patient care can exacerbate resistance to change.

STRATEGIES TO ADDRESS RESISTANCE

A. Communication and Engagement: Transparent, consistent communication helps build trust and reduce uncertainty.

- **Articulate the Vision**: Clearly explain the purpose and benefits of the transformation, emphasizing its alignment with organizational goals and the improvement of patient care.

- **Two-Way Communication**: Establish platforms for stakeholders to voice concerns and provide feedback, such as town halls or digital surveys.
- **Engage Early and Often**: Involve key stakeholders from the diagnostic phase to foster ownership and reduce resistance.

B. Leadership and Role Modeling: Leadership plays a pivotal role in overcoming resistance by setting the tone for change.

- **Visible Commitment**: Senior leaders should actively support the change initiative through consistent messaging and actions.
- **Change Champions**: Identify and empower influential employees to advocate for the transformation.
- **Empathy and Support**: Leaders must acknowledge the emotional aspects of change and provide reassurance.

C. Tailored Training and Resources: Resistance often arises from a lack of confidence or knowledge about new processes or technologies.

- **Comprehensive Training Programs**: Tailor training to address the specific needs of each role.
- **Continuous Support**: Offer resources, such as help desks or on-the-job coaching, to facilitate a smooth transition.
- **Focus on Quick Wins**: Demonstrate early successes to build momentum and reinforce commitment.

MITIGATING SYSTEMIC BARRIERS

A. Cultural Transformation

- **Assess Organizational Culture**: Identify aspects of the culture that may resist change and align initiatives to address these challenges.

- **Promote a Growth Mindset**: Encourage an organizational attitude that views change as an opportunity rather than a threat.

B. Flexible Implementation

- **Pilot Programs**: Test changes on a smaller scale before full implementation to identify and address potential challenges.
- **Iterative Adjustments**: Utilize feedback to refine processes and ensure they align with the organization's diverse needs.

C. Resource Allocation

- Ensure that adequate resources, including staffing, technology, and funding, are available to support the transition.
- Address workload concerns by redistributing tasks or providing additional support during the transition.

Addressing Resistance in Specific Stakeholder Groups

A. Physicians and Clinical Staff

- Highlight the impact on patient outcomes, a core motivator for clinicians.
- Involve them in decision-making processes to ensure the transformation aligns with clinical priorities.

B. Administrative Staff

- Emphasize operational efficiencies and career development opportunities that arise from the transformation.
- Provide clear guidelines and robust training to facilitate a smooth transition.

C. Patients

- Educate patients on how the changes will improve their care experience.
- Use patient advocates to build trust and credibility within the community.

Measuring Success in Addressing Resistance
- **Adoption Rates**: The percentage of staff utilizing new systems or processes.
- **Engagement Levels**: Staff participation in training and feedback sessions.
- **Performance Indicators**: Improvements in patient outcomes, operational efficiency, or satisfaction scores.
- **Feedback Analysis**: Regular surveys to gauge stakeholder sentiment and identify lingering resistance.

Resistance to change is an inevitable aspect of transformation in healthcare. By understanding the sector's unique challenges and employing targeted strategies, healthcare leaders can minimize resistance and ensure the success of change initiatives.

Transparent communication, empathetic leadership, and a culture of collaboration are key to overcoming barriers and driving sustainable transformation.

CASE STUDY: CONTEXT – DRIVEN TRANSFORMATION AT APOLLO HOSPITALS AND LV PRASAD EYE INSTITUTE

Apollo Hospitals and the LV Prasad Eye Institute (LVPEI) are exemplary cases of healthcare organizations in India that have successfully implemented transformation strategies tailored to their specific contexts.

Apollo Hospitals
Founded in 1983 by Dr. Prathap C. Reddy, Apollo Hospitals has grown into one of Asia's largest and most trusted healthcare providers. Over the past four decades, the organization has undergone significant transformations to adapt to the evolving healthcare landscape.

Key strategies include:

- **Expansion and Diversification**: Apollo Hospitals has expanded its footprint across India and internationally, establishing a network of hospitals, clinics, pharmacies, and diagnostic centers. This extensive network ensures accessibility to quality healthcare services for a broad population.
- **Technological Integration**: The organization has been at the forefront of adopting advanced medical technologies, including robotic surgeries, telemedicine, and electronic health records. These innovations have enhanced patient care, operational efficiency, and clinical outcomes.
- **Emphasize Preventive Healthcare**: Recognizing the importance of preventive care, Apollo Hospitals has introduced initiatives such as health check-up packages and wellness programs to facilitate early detection and management of diseases.
- **Public-Private Partnerships**: Apollo has collaborated with various state governments in India to manage public hospitals and provide quality healthcare services, leveraging its expertise to support the public sector.
- **Educational Initiatives**: Through the Apollo Hospitals Educational and Research Foundation, the organization has contributed to the development of healthcare professionals by offering a range of medical and paramedical courses.
- **Digital Health Platforms**: In response to the digital revolution, Apollo has developed platforms like Apollo 24/7, which provide online consultations, medicine delivery, and health record management, thereby enhancing patient engagement and accessibility.

LV Prasad Eye Institute (LVPEI): Established in 1987 by Dr. Gullapalli N. Rao, LVPEI has emerged as a world-class eye care institution dedicated to comprehensive patient care, clinical research, and education. Its transformation strategies include:

- **Comprehensive Eye Care Model**: LVPEI operates on a pyramidal model, with tertiary centers at the top, secondary centers in districts, and primary care centers in rural areas. This structure ensures that eye care services are accessible to urban and rural populations.

- **Focus on Research and Innovation**: The institute emphasizes research in ophthalmology, contributing to advancements in eye care. It has developed cost-effective solutions and innovative products, such as the award-winning visual field screening device Order of Magnitude (OM), which has screened over 100,000 eyes.

- **Capacity Building and Training**: LVPEI has trained numerous eye care professionals, including ophthalmologists, optometrists, and support staff, strengthening the eye care workforce in India and other developing countries.

- **Community Engagement:** The institute actively engages with communities through outreach programs, eye donation drives, and awareness campaigns, fostering a culture of eye health consciousness.

- **Sustainability and Accessibility**: LVPEI provides over 50% of its services free of cost to economically underprivileged patients, ensuring equitable access to eye care.

- **Technological Advancements**: The institute has developed in-house technologies, such as the PROSE lens in collaboration with the Boston Foundation for Sight, USA, to treat complex corneal conditions, and the ConnectCare app-based teleconsultation service, which enabled over 50,000 patient consultations, saving about INR 60 million in travel costs and reducing carbon emissions.

Both Apollo Hospitals and LVPEI have demonstrated that a clear vision, commitment to quality, and adaptability to changing environments are crucial for successful transformation in the healthcare sector.

Their strategies offer valuable insights for other organizations implementing context-specific transformation initiatives.

CASE STUDY: AYUSHMAN BHARAT DIGITAL MISSION – A NATIONAL-LEVEL DIGITAL HEALTH TRANSFORMATION IN INDIA

India's healthcare system, vast in scale and diversity, has historically grappled with fragmented data systems, inefficiencies, and inequitable access to care. In response to these challenges, the Ayushman Bharat Digital Mission (ABDM) was launched on September 27, 2021, under the National Health Authority (NHA) of the Ministry of Health and Family Welfare.

The program set forth an ambitious goal: to create an integrated digital health ecosystem that improves efficiency, transparency, and accessibility in healthcare delivery nationwide. ABDM aims to unify stakeholders—including patients, healthcare providers, insurers, and technology vendors—through interoperable digital platforms while ensuring individual privacy, equity, and data security.

The initiative is rooted in a patient-centric philosophy, emphasizing empowerment through digital health accounts and transparent consent management systems.

Strategic Objectives and Vision: The core objectives of ABDM include:

- Universal access to digital healthcare, irrespective of geography or socioeconomic status.
- Interoperable infrastructure through standardized digital health records and systems.

- Empowerment of individuals via Ayushman Bharat Health Accounts (ABHA) that link personal health data across public and private systems.
- Integration of health professionals and facilities into national registries, ensuring standardized service quality.
- Data-driven policymaking allows for real-time trend analysis and responsive interventions.

Implementation Strategy and Leadership Approach: ABDM's rollout followed a phased and iterative change management model, emphasizing strategic planning, stakeholder engagement, and robust monitoring and evaluation.

- **Infrastructure Development**: A foundational effort involved creating digital registries of patients (ABHA IDs), professionals (Healthcare Professionals Registry, HPR), and facilities (Health Facility Registry, HFR). These platforms ensured data portability, increased transparency, and set the stage for interoperability.
- **Stakeholder Collaboration and Onboarding**: The NHA led extensive collaboration efforts across the public and private sectors. Healthcare institutions, technology firms, insurers, and diagnostic providers were systematically onboarded, supported by technical resources and incentives.
- **Microsite Launches and Pilot Programs**: Pilot projects, such as QR-code-based OPD registrations, were initiated through microsites in various districts to test the feasibility of digital processes. These implementations informed broader national scaling strategies.
- **Incentive Mechanisms**: The Digital Health Incentive Scheme (DHIS) was introduced to accelerate the adoption of digital health solutions.

Financial incentives encouraged private sector participation, particularly in underserved and rural areas.

- **Digital Service Expansion**: Telehealth services, such as eSanjeevani, were integrated to provide remote consultation options. These innovations proved vital in enhancing rural healthcare delivery.

Outcomes and Impact: In just over three years, the ABDM has demonstrated measurable progress:

- 67 crore ABHA IDs were generated, providing individuals with portable, accessible digital health records.
- 42 crore health records have been digitally linked, facilitating seamless care across facilities.
- Over 3.3 lakh health facilities and 4.7 lakh healthcare professionals have been integrated into the system.
- Participation from 236 private entities, including laboratories and pharmacies, has strengthened the program's scalability and relevance.
- Flagship institutions, such as AIIMS Delhi and Bhopal, have successfully operationalized ABDM features, modeling best practices in digital transformation.
- These results reflect a significant shift toward a unified and efficient healthcare infrastructure that can support real-time care coordination and policy design.

Challenges and Barriers to Change: Despite notable success, ABDM has encountered substantial challenges that required strategic leadership and adaptive change management:

- **Digital Infrastructure Gaps**: Limited internet penetration and connectivity in rural areas posed significant hurdles for onboarding and implementation.

- **Resistance to Change**: Many healthcare professionals and institutions have demonstrated reluctance to shift from legacy systems to digital workflows, driven by concerns about usability, training, and the fear of disruption.
- **Privacy and Data Security**: Public trust was tested by concerns regarding the misuse of health data. Compliance with the Digital Personal Data Protection Act, 2023, was crucial in mitigating this risk.
- **Regulatory Ambiguities**: Questions surrounding data ownership, consent mechanisms, and third-party vendor accountability created operational uncertainty.

Leadership and Change Management Insights

The ABDM's journey reflects a pragmatic and responsive approach to national-level transformation. Key leadership and change management strategies include:

- **Visionary Framing**: Clear articulation of long-term goals, such as improved access and equity, built widespread support, and aligned stakeholders.
- **Empowering Stakeholders:** By involving healthcare professionals in training and offering digital literacy support, leaders reduced resistance and facilitated smoother transitions.
- **Iterative Implementation:** Pilot programs were used to gather feedback and optimize technical frameworks before scaling.
- **Trust Building Through Transparency**: A robust consent architecture and clear communication around data usage helped establish credibility.
- **Policy-Driven Change**: Regulatory alignment and incentivization schemes facilitated compliance and sustained engagement, particularly among private sector actors.

Lessons Learned: ABDM's case offers several transferable lessons for healthcare transformation globally:

- Infrastructure investment is foundational. Digital health ecosystems cannot thrive without reliable connectivity and access to hardware.
- Stakeholder engagement is non-negotiable. Change is most effective when it is participatory, not prescriptive.
- Security and privacy must be central, not peripheral. Building trust requires robust safeguards and transparent processes.
- An iterative, learning-based approach enhances adoption. Flexibility and feedback mechanisms are key to sustainable reform.

The Ayushman Bharat Digital Mission represents a pioneering effort to digitize healthcare on a national scale in a diverse and populous country. It stands as a case study in effective public sector leadership, thoughtful change management, and inclusive design. While challenges remain, ABDM has set a global precedent in leveraging digital technology to enhance healthcare equity, efficiency, and empowerment.

If India can address the remaining gaps—particularly those related to infrastructure, stakeholder alignment, and regulatory clarity—it is poised to establish a resilient, tech-enabled healthcare system for the 21st century.

References

1. NHA | Official website Ayushman Bharat Digital Mission [Internet]. [cited 2024 Dec 6]. Available from: https://abdm.gov.in/abdm-components
2. Ayushman Bharat Digital Mission (ABDM) | Health-e [Internet]. 2023 [cited 2024 Dec 4].
2. Available from: https://health-e.in/blog/abdm/
3. Ayushman Bharat Digital Mission marks a Transformative Three-Year Journey towards enabling Digital Health | Ministry of Health and Family Welfare |

GOI [Internet]. [cited 2024 Nov 14]. Available from: https://www.mohfw.gov.in/?q=pressrelease-87

4. Sapnani S. Challenges in Creating a Unified Health Record System in India: A Focus on "ABHA."

5. operational_Guidelines_9d3cf828f4.pdf [Internet]. [cited 2024 Dec 5]. Available from: https://abdm.gov.in:8081/uploads/operational_Guidelin es_9d3cf828f4.pdf

6. Drishti IAS [Internet]. [cited 2024 Dec 5]. 3 Years of Ayushman Bharat Digital Mission. Available from: https://www.drishtiias.com/daily-updates/daily-news-analysis/3-years-of-ayushman-bharat-digital-mission

7. Ayushman Bharat Digital Mission: Boon or Bane? [Internet]. Accountability Initiative: Responsive Governance. [cited 2024 Dec 5]. Available from: https://accountabilityindia.in/blog/ayushman-bharat-digital-mission-boon-or-bane/

8. Hindustan Times [Internet]. 2024 [cited 2024 Dec 5]. Impact of Ayushman Bharat Digital Mission (ABDM). Available from: https://www.hindustantimes.com/ht-insight/public-health/impact-of-ayushman-bharat-digital-mission-abdm-101725259895868.html

9. Mishra US, Yadav S, Joe W. The Ayushman Bharat Digital Mission of India: An Assessment. Health Systems & Reform. 2024 Dec 17;10(2):2392290.

10. Overcoming Challenges in ABDM Integration | LinkedIn [Internet]. [cited 2024 Dec 5]. Available from: https://www.linkedin.com/pulse/overcoming-challenges-abdm-integration-bluebashco-zdajc/

11. ABDM-Report.pdf [Internet]. [cited 2024 Dec 5]. Available from: https://www.rich.telangana.gov.in/assets/pdfs/Reports/ABDM-Report.pdf

12. Athaley C. Ayushman Bharat Digital Mission - India's Leapfrog Moment.

POLICY TO ACTION CASE STUDY IN DISCUSSION WITH FARHAD ALI: CALORIE LABELING IN RESTAURANTS – QUEZON CITY, PHILIPPINES

This case study presents the experience of implementing a calorie labeling policy in Quezon City, Philippines. The insights and reflections are drawn from a comprehensive conversation with **Farhad Ali**, a key practitioner who led the initiative, navigating technical, legal, and political complexities on the ground.

Policy Objective: To combat rising obesity and non-communicable diseases (NCDs) in Quezon City by mandating calorie information on menus in chain restaurants, empowering consumers to make informed food choices. The municipal corporation and the Mayor were keenly involved and driving the initiative.

1. **Context & Background**
   - **Public Health Concern**: Sharp rise in obesity, diabetes, and hypertension, especially among urban working youth.
   - **Social Norms**: Eating out is a common, affordable, and socially accepted practice, particularly among migrants and working-class youth.
   - **Key Locations**: Chain restaurants such as McDonald's, Jollibee, KFC.
2. **Intervention Design**
   - **Policy Focus**: Mandate visible calorie labeling on restaurant menus.
   - **Scientific Basis**: Evidence suggests that visibility of calorie information reduces caloric intake and pushes businesses to offer healthier options.
   - **Implementation Phases**: Multiple phases targeting restaurants based on scale and reach.
3. **Local Context Analysis**
   - **Cultural Practices**: High external food consumption due to affordability and convenience.

- **Existing Data**: Supported by local surveys and health department data on NCD prevalence and dietary habits.

4. **Stakeholder Engagement**
   - **Key Stakeholders:**
     - Municipal Corporation
     - Mayor's Office
     - Health & Nutrition Department
     - Business & Licensing Department
     - Legal Department
     - Restaurant Chains
   - **Stakeholder Management Strategies:**
     - Building rapport through ongoing engagement.
     - Ensuring mayoral visibility and commitment, a key person driving the initiative
     - Aligning policy goals with departmental mandates.
     - Addressing industry pushback (e.g., resistance to display vs QR code) through legal and technical reasoning.

5. **Policy Development Challenges**
   - **Industry Pushback**: Attempts to dilute the policy with QR code suggestions.
   - **Bureaucratic Complexities**: Interdepartmental power struggles and delays in signing legal agreements.
   - **Technical Hurdles**: Ensuring accuracy in calorie data, certifying labs, and legal enforcement authority.

6. **Enablers of Change**
   - **Strong Political Will**: Committed leadership from
   - the mayor who sought legacy-driven reform.
   - **Technical Expertise**: Partnerships with legal firms and nutritional experts.
   - **Capacity Building**: Development of manuals, M&E tools, IT tracking systems, and department-level training.

7. **Monitoring & Evaluation**
   - **Framework Developed**: Includes behavioral surveys, restaurant menu audits, and health impact indicators.

- **Ownership Transfer Plan**: Local government to take over post-project; tools, frameworks, and IT systems to be handed over.
- **Timeframe**: Long-term M&E over 3–5 years post-implementation.

8. **Sustainability Measures**
   - Training across municipal departments.
   - System-level reforms and digital tools to institutionalize enforcement.
   - Public campaigns to maintain awareness and demand.
   - Integration into larger global networks (e.g., Partnership for Healthy Cities).

9. **Lessons & Reflections**
   - **Adaptive Management**: Fixed systems often failed under real-time conditions. Leadership team was flexible and adaptive to the requirements of the stakeholders for successful policy implementation
   - **Persistence Pays**: Constant engagement, even during bureaucratic deadlocks, was crucial.
   - **Systems Thinking**: Building Ecosystems for Change—Beyond Policy Text—Ensures Long-Term Sustainability.

This case illustrates how strategic alignment, political commitment, and community-informed design can turn a simple policy idea into a scalable public health intervention. It also underscores the need for systemic change and institutional resilience to achieve long-term success.

CASE STUDY: EGYPT'S HEPATITIS C ELIMINATION PROGRAM – A NATIONAL HEALTH TRANSFORMATION

Egypt once had one of the highest global burdens of Hepatitis C Virus (HCV), with a 2015 prevalence estimated at 6% and associated mortality accounting for over 18,000 deaths annually. To address this national crisis, the Egyptian government, through the

National Committee for Control of Viral Hepatitis (NCCVH), launched an ambitious program in 2014 aimed at eliminating HCV. This initiative evolved into one of the most comprehensive, government-led public health campaigns globally, aligning with the World Health Organization (WHO) targets for hepatitis elimination.

The transformation centered on a strategy of mass screening, accessible and affordable treatment using Direct-Acting Antivirals (DAAs), and robust infection control, all underpinned by political will, innovative financing, and technological integration.

Strategic Vision and Implementation Framework

The government's vision was to reduce HCV-related morbidity and mortality, aiming for elimination by 2023. The strategy was guided by the Egyptian Viral Hepatitis Action Plan (2014), which laid out a holistic framework comprising:

- **Comprehensive Screening and Diagnosis**: Under the "100 million Healthy Lives" campaign, more than 60 million Egyptians were screened for HCV, diabetes, and hypertension between 2018 and 2019. Rapid Diagnostic Tests (RDTs) enabled same-day results, particularly benefiting rural and underserved populations.
- **Affordable and Scalable Treatment Rollout**: In 2014, Egypt transitioned from expensive and less effective interferon-based therapies to direct-acting antivirals (DAAs). The government negotiated with Gilead Sciences to reduce the cost of sofosbuvir from $28,000 to $300, and subsequently enabled the local production of generics, reducing the treatment cost to under $100 per course. Over 100 treatment centers were established, supported by a centralized online registration platform.
- **Public Awareness and Stigma Reduction**: National media campaigns, community health worker outreach, and culturally tailored messaging were deployed to overcome stigma and misinformation. Emphasis was placed on early diagnosis, curative potential, and prevention.

- **Technological Integration and Data Analytics**: Web-based registration systems and epidemiological data platforms streamlined treatment assignment, enabled real-time tracking, and informed policy decisions. These tools also improved accountability and resource allocation.
- **Innovative Financing and Global Partnerships**: The Egyptian government secured $250 million from the World Bank and allocated significant national resources. This multi-source financing model ensured free screening and treatment for all citizens.
- **Monitoring and Evaluation**: Regular assessments, patient satisfaction surveys, and health worker feedback loops allowed iterative improvement and adaptability. Surveillance systems tracked prevalence, reinfection rates, and treatment outcomes.

Outcomes and Impact: By 2023, the program had achieved transformative outcomes:
- Over 4.1 million individuals treated with cure rates above 95% (sustained virologic response).
- Prevalence reduced from 6% (2015) to 0.5%, meeting WHO Gold Tier elimination status.
- An estimated 250,000 deaths and 150,000 cases of liver cancer were prevented.
- $557 million investment yielded projected savings of $7 billion through reduced long-term complications.

Challenges and Barriers: Despite its success, the initiative encountered significant hurdles:
- **Initial Treatment Limitations**: Early therapies such as PEG-RBV were costly, less effective (27–45% cure rate), and had severe side effects, leading to patient dropout.
- **Infrastructure Gaps**: Rural areas initially lacked screening centers and diagnostic equipment.
- **Stigma and Misinformation**: Cultural Misconceptions

about HCV Transmission Inhibit Community Engagement.

- **Financial Constraints**: As a middle-income country, Egypt had to find innovative ways to fund a population-wide health initiative.
- **Genotype Challenges**: Most global antiviral regimens were initially ineffective against Egypt's dominant HCV genotype 4, necessitating targeted research and development efforts, as well as customized therapy protocols.

Leadership and Change Management: Strong leadership and adaptive change management were at the heart of the program's success:

- **High-Level Political Commitment**: The Egyptian President and the Ministry of Health have made HCV elimination a national priority, ensuring sustained visibility and funding.
- **Centralized Strategic Coordination**: The NCCVH led national efforts with a clear governance framework, integrating ministries, health professionals, and global partners to achieve a unified approach.
- **Negotiation and Innovation**: Egyptian leadership secured reduced pricing, IP concessions, and local manufacturing through effective public-private engagement.
- **Decentralized Execution**: Regional centers were empowered to adapt and implement programs in context-specific ways, thereby enhancing responsiveness.
- **Technological Leverage**: Digital tools enabled real-time data use, streamlined registration, and optimized decision-making.

Lessons Learned: Key insights from Egypt's program that are transferable to other healthcare transformation efforts include:

- **Visionary Leadership Enables Scale**: Sustained high-level political support was crucial for mobilizing resources and overcoming inertia.
- **Affordability is Foundational**: Local drug manufacturing and global partnerships made large-scale treatment feasible.
- **Technology is a Catalyst**: Digital platforms reduce delays, improve efficiency, and enable evidence-based adjustments.
- **Inclusivity Ensures Impact**: Reaching marginalized and rural populations ensured equity and effectiveness.
- **Iterative Feedback Loops Matter**: Monitoring and stakeholder engagement improved program design and outcomes over time.

Egypt's HCV elimination initiative is a landmark in the global transformation of health. Through a powerful combination of political will, inclusive policy, technological innovation, and international collaboration, the country successfully addressed one of its most pressing public health challenges.

The program treated millions, saved billions in future costs, and built health infrastructure that will serve beyond HCV elimination. This case offers a replicable model for other low- and middle-income countries seeking to achieve the WHO's health targets. It demonstrates that with strategic leadership, cross-sectoral partnerships, and patient-centered design, even the most ambitious health reforms are attainable.

References

1. WHO commends Egypt for its progress on the path to eliminate hepatitis C [Internet]. [cited 2024 Oct 30]. Available from: https://www.who.int/news/item/09-10-2023-who-commends-egypt-for-its-progress-on-the-path-to-eliminate-hepatitis-c.

2. National Hepatitis Elimination Profile-Egypt-March1.pdf [Internet]. [cited 2024 Oct 30]. Available from: https://www.globalhep.org/sites/default/files/content/page/files/2022-08/National%20Hepatitis%20Elimination%20Profile-Egypt-March1.pdf

3. Egyptian Viral Hepatitis Action Plan 2014.pdf [Internet]. [cited 2024 Oct 30]. Available from: https://www.globalhep.org/sites/default/files/content/action_plan_article/files/2020-04/Egyptian%20Viral%20Hepatitis%20Action%20Plan%202014.pdf

4. World Bank [Internet]. [cited 2024 Oct 30]. How Egypt Won Its Battle Against Hepatitis C. Available from: https://www.worldbank.org/en/news/feature/2024/04/05/how-egypt-won-its-battle-against-hepatitis-c

5. Gomaa A, Gomaa M, Allam N, Waked I. Hepatitis C Elimination in Egypt: Story of Success. Pathogens. 2024 Aug;13(8):681.

6. WEF_The_Art_and_Science_of_Eliminating_Hepatitis_Egypt's_Experience_2022.pdf [Internet]. [cited 2024 Oct 30]. Available from: https://www3.weforum.org/docs/WEF_The_Art_and_Science_of_Eliminating_Hepatitis_Egypts_Experience_2022.pdf

7. Hassanin A, Kamel S, Waked I, Fort M. Egypt's Ambitious Strategy to Eliminate Hepatitis C Virus: A Case Study. Glob Health Sci Pract. 2021 Mar 31;9(1):187–200.

8. Waked I. Case study of hepatitis C virus control in Egypt: impact of access program. Antivir Ther. 2022 Apr;27(2):13596535211067592.

CASE STUDY: LEADERSHIP LESSONS IN HEALTHCARE TRANSFORMATION – A CONVERSATION WITH DR. HALA ZAID, FORMER MINISTER OF HEALTH AND POPULATION, EGYPT

Dr. Hala Zaid served as Egypt's Minister of Health and Population during one of the most transformative periods in the country's healthcare history. Under her leadership, Egypt implemented the Hepatitis C elimination program, initiated public health campaigns, established the Egyptian Drug Authority, the Universal Health Insurance Authority, and the Unified Purchasing Agency, and managed the COVID-19 pandemic response.

Her leadership journey offers profound insights into change management, systems thinking, and the sustainability of reforms.

This case study is based on an in-depth conversation with Dr. Zaid, who reflects on her leadership approach, the challenges she faces, and the strategies she employs to sustain transformative change in a complex health system.

Vision-Driven but Adaptive Leadership

Dr. Zaid emphasized that effective leadership requires a balance between vision and adaptability. She stated:

"You must remain focused on your goals, but if the external environment changes, you need to be flexible. Don't resist change—respond to it wisely."

Her approach involved setting clear objectives but being open to modifying them in response to external shocks, such as political shifts or health crises. She also stressed that leaders must align their ambitions with institutional missions:

"It's dangerous to lead based on your personal vision. Serve the organization's vision; personal achievements will follow."

Investing in Human Capital for Sustainability

Sustainability, according to Dr. Zaid, is not about systems alone—it is about people:

"The only sustainable way is to invest in human resources."

She spearheaded partnerships with institutions like Harvard Medical School to train more than 4000 Egyptian healthcare professionals in global health, quality management, and leadership. These trained individuals now occupy top positions in Egypt's public health system. She institutionalized change by embedding initiatives, such as those in the public health sector, into the ministry's formal structure, ensuring continuity beyond her tenure.

The Hepatitis C Program – A Leadership Blueprint

Dr. Zaid's leadership of the 100 million Healthy Lives campaign illustrates her strategic and people-centered approach to change. She:

- Selected technical experts with strong ethical values to lead the campaign.
- Met daily with teams, transferring knowledge and empowering them.
- Created formal mechanisms for communication, tracking progress through flipcharts in her office.
- Delivered screening and treatment to over 60 million people in 7 months.

She noted: ***"The success of Hepatitis C elimination wasn't just medical. It was organizational, political, and human."***

She cultivated second-line leaders and evaluated their performance not just by results, but also by their ability to build sustainable teams.

Change Management and Resistance

Dr. Zaid faced significant resistance—not from within her ministry, but from other ministries essential to health reform (e.g., Finance, Planning, Social Solidarity). To manage this, she leveraged presidential support and clear, public accountability.

"Without support from the President, my effort would have led to zero outcome."

She also adopted a sense of urgency by committing publicly to bold targets—e.g., screening 70 million Egyptians in 7 months—thus galvanizing her team and aligning stakeholders.

Empowerment and Institutionalization

A key tenet of Dr. Zaid's change management approach was empowerment without blame: *"Don't blame people. Empower them. If someone doesn't respond, try again. If needed, change them—but only after multiple trials of support."*

She advocated for the institutionalization of reforms by restructuring ministries and creating new independent authorities like the Egyptian Drug Authority, while maintaining respect for senior officials:

Cross-Sector Collaboration and System Integration:
Understanding that health outcomes rely on intersectoral coordination, Dr. Zaid:

- Formed inter-agency committees with heads of various health authorities.
- Shared Ministry of Health budgets with university hospitals (under the Ministry of Higher Education) to support public health outcomes.
- Engaged the private sector during the pandemic, providing free access to critical medicines and equipment to hospitals treating COVID-19 patients. She explained: *"People don't care if the hospital is public or private. When someone dies, they blame the Ministry of Health. So, I had to support them all."*

Learning-Oriented Leadership

Dr. Zaid underscored the importance of lifelong learning and experience-based training. She highlighted a leadership course at Harvard that had a lasting impact because it blended theory with peer learning and real-world problem-solving.

She argued against purely theoretical training and suggested: *"Invite both successful and failed leaders to share their experiences. You can learn from both success and failure."*

She also implemented mentorship and coaching systems within the ministry, believing that leaders should remain accessible to their teams beyond the classroom.

Succession Planning and Cultural Transformation

Institutionalizing change, according to Dr. Zaid, meant cultivating a culture of shared leadership and succession readiness. She reviewed team members not just for their achievements, but for whether they had prepared the next generation of leaders.

"A strong leader creates strong leaders. If your team collapses after you leave, then you failed."

She used structured delegation, respect for elders, and value alignment as tools to reduce resistance and instill continuity in leadership pipelines. Dr. Hala Zaid's leadership journey illustrates a comprehensive and human-centered model of healthcare transformation. Her ability to combine vision with responsiveness, emphasize education and empowerment, and institutionalize reform efforts through strategic alliances and structured change management makes her a compelling example of transformational leadership in global health.

Her advice to future leaders: *"Be patient-focused. Any decision that doesn't improve lives is not worth taking. Empower your people. Listen more. Blame less. That's the only way to build sustainable systems."*

CASE STUDY: REFLECTIONS ON LEADERSHIP AND SUSTAINABILITY IN PUBLIC HEALTH — A CONVERSATION WITH FARHAD ALI

In the rapidly evolving world of public health, leadership is often exercised not solely through authority but through a clarity of vision, adaptability, and thoughtful engagement with systems and people. Farhad Ali, a senior public health professional with decades of experience across Asia, Southeast Asia, and Africa, reflects on his journey of designing and managing healthcare initiatives, particularly in challenging environments. This case study, based on a conversation for the Leadership and Change Management (LCM) book, distills his experiences into practical insights for emerging leaders in healthcare.

Motivation and Organizational Culture

Ali begins by discussing motivation in public health work. While financial incentives are often seen as primary drivers, he emphasizes the power of non-financial motivators, such as staff recognition, acknowledgment of contributions, and institutional policies that value people.

"Financial incentives definitely work, but non-financial incentives—like public recognition, appreciation by leadership, and internal culture—can be just as powerful."

He argues that leadership must intentionally cultivate a culture of motivation by embedding recognition mechanisms into organizational processes.

Defining and Designing for Sustainability

A central theme in the conversation is sustainability—a term frequently used but rarely defined precisely in public health.

Ali offers a nuanced perspective:

- Sustainability must be defined explicitly—whether it refers to sustaining project outcomes, organizational practices, or institutional capacity.

- He challenges the notion of indefinite continuity, proposing that leaders instead define how long something should be sustained and who will carry it forward.

"Nothing is sustainable forever. You must ask: do we need to sustain this for six months, two years, or ten years? Then design accordingly."

He draws inspiration from public-private partnership models, where one entity builds a program and another manages or sustains it after transition.

The Limits of Sustainability: A Realistic Lens

Ali provides a candid critique of the often-romanticized idea of sustainable health programs. Using the polio eradication campaign as an example, he highlights the mismatch between stated goals and ongoing realities.

"The goal was to eradicate polio so the program could end. But even after eradication, vaccination campaigns continue. So, is that success or failure? We must be honest in how we define and measure sustainability."

He shares an example from a childhood diarrhea management project, where success was measured not by institutional continuity, but by whether mothers could correctly identify symptoms and access a trained community health worker. This human-centered metric, he argues, reflects deeper sustainability than any log frame indicator.

Training, Mentoring, and Leadership Development

Ali reflects critically on the role of training in leadership development:

"Training is helpful—but only when given to the right people at the right time."

He believes that exposure to real-world problems is essential for practical leadership training. Without context, training remains theoretical. Case studies rooted in local settings—rather than imported from the West—are essential for relevance and resonance.

- Ali is a strong advocate of mentoring and coaching as long-term strategies for leadership development.

"As leaders grow, they must learn to question their own beliefs. Mentors help us stay grounded, reflective, and open to change."

- He emphasizes that leadership development must include space for doubt, dialogue, and reflection—not just tools and checklists.

Organizational Culture and Change: When discussing how change can be managed within institutions, Ali emphasizes the use of observation as a diagnostic tool for effective management. He encourages new leaders to pay attention to the discrepancy between stated values and lived experiences:

"You'll hear about values in your orientation, but the real culture is what you observe—how supervisors act, how decisions are made, and how staff are supported."

This distinction between espoused values and operational realities is crucial for assessing an organization's readiness for change. On working across silos, he notes that while some degree of siloed work is inevitable, many health challenges today—such as non-communicable diseases—require cross-sectoral collaboration:

"If you're working on diabetes, you need expertise in urban design, air quality, food systems, and communications. No single unit can hold all that."

Advice for Emerging Leaders: Ali offers candid guidance for young professionals tasked with driving change in challenging environments:

- Don't try to overhaul systems on day one.
- First, establish credibility by delivering on core responsibilities.
- Then use informal channels—like conversations over tea—to build rapport and influence.

"Demonstrate your value first. Be practical. Change is easier when people trust your ability to deliver."

He also emphasizes the importance of timing and receptivity. Proposing significant changes during organizational stress or external crises often backfires. Leaders must be attuned to organizational rhythm and readiness.

Farhad Ali's reflections offer a grounded and humanistic perspective on leadership in public health. His approach blends systems thinking with cultural sensitivity, strategic patience with pragmatic execution. For mid-career professionals, his insights underscore that effective leadership is not about charisma or position—it's about contextual intelligence, personal humility, and an unwavering commitment to people.

"Vision is important. But to get there, the path won't be straight. You'll walk in curves, adapt, pivot. That's what leadership really is."

DIAGNOSTIC PHASE

Identifying the distinct needs of a healthcare environment before enacting transformation strategies is essential for aligning the transformation with the setting's unique traits and challenges. This stage, known as the diagnostic phase, involves a systematic approach to collecting insights, assessing the current situation, and developing strategic initiatives tailored to the specific context.

Key Steps in the Diagnostic Phase
1. Assessment of Current State

- **Recognizing Organizational Aims**: Determine the primary goals of the healthcare organization, such as enhancing patient outcomes, improving operational efficiency, or increasing access to services.
- **Mapping Current Operations**: Document existing workflows, resource utilization, patient pathways, and

service delivery models to identify areas for improvement and optimization.

- **Engaging Stakeholders**: Collaborate with internal stakeholders (e.g., clinicians and administrators) and external stakeholders (e.g., patients and policymakers) to understand their perspectives and identify their key concerns and pain points.
- **Data Collection and Analysis**: Use quantitative data (e.g., patient outcomes, financial reports, operational metrics) and qualitative insights (e.g., staff feedback, patient satisfaction surveys) to establish a baseline understanding.

2. Understanding the Healthcare Landscape

- **Regulatory and Policy Environment**: Analyze compliance requirements, accreditation standards, and national or regional healthcare policies.
- **Patient Demographics and Needs**: Examine the population served, focusing on factors such as age distribution, socioeconomic status, disease prevalence, and cultural considerations.
- **Technological Readiness**: Assess the organization's current technology infrastructure and readiness to adopt new digital tools or systems.

3. Identifying Gaps and Opportunities

- **Gap Analysis**: Compare the current state with desired outcomes to identify areas needing improvement, such as inefficiencies, resource shortages, or outdated practices.
- **Opportunity Mapping**: Highlight potential areas for innovation, such as leveraging telemedicine, adopting value-based care models, or integrating artificial intelligence in diagnostics.

4. Strategic Alignment

- **Prioritization of Needs**: Categorize identified needs into short-term and long-term priorities based on urgency, feasibility, and impact.
- **Stakeholder Buy-In**: Ensure alignment among leadership, staff, and external stakeholders to build consensus on the identified needs and proposed changes.

5. Risk Assessment

- **Identifying Barriers**: Pinpoint potential resistance to change, resource limitations, and operational disruptions that could arise during implementation.
- **Developing Mitigation Strategies**: Plan for addressing these challenges through effective communication, training, and resource allocation.

Frameworks and Tools for the Diagnostic Phase: Healthcare organizations often employ specific frameworks and tools during the diagnostic phase to structure their analyses and ensure comprehensive assessments.

1. SWOT Analysis

- **Strengths**: Identify internal assets, such as skilled personnel, advanced equipment, or strong leadership.
- **Weaknesses**: Pinpoint internal limitations, such as outdated processes or staff shortages.
- **Opportunities**: Recognize external growth possibilities, such as government funding or emerging technologies.
- **Threats**: Assess external risks, including regulatory changes and competition.

2. Stakeholder Analysis: Identify key stakeholders, their roles, and their level of influence within the organization. Identify champions for the transformation initiative and potential opponents.

3. Root Cause Analysis: Utilize tools such as Fishbone Diagrams or the Five Whys method to investigate the root causes of identified issues.

4. Process Mapping: Create visual representations of workflows to identify bottlenecks, redundancies,or inefficiencies.

Leadership in the Diagnostic Phase: Effective leadership plays a pivotal role in navigating the diagnostic phase. Leaders must:

- **Communicate a Clear Vision**: Articulate the purpose and potential benefits of the transformation to all stakeholders.
- **Foster Collaboration**: Build interdisciplinary teams that include clinical, administrative, and technical experts.
- **Promote Transparency**: Share findings and progress with stakeholders to build trust and engagement.
- **Encourage Innovation**: Create an environment where team members feel empowered to propose creative solutions.

Strategic Thinking and Design: After completing the diagnostic phase, organizations proceed to design strategic initiatives. This involves:

- **Defining Clear Objectives**: Establish specific, measurable, achievable, relevant, and time-bound (SMART) goals for the transformation.
- **Developing Action Plans**: Break down objectives into actionable steps, assigning responsibilities and timelines to ensure effective implementation.
- **Allocating Resources**: Identify and secure the financial, human, and technological resources needed for implementation.

For example, a public health program aiming to reduce maternal mortality might develop initiatives such as:

- Training midwives in rural areas to improve skilled birth attendance (short-term goals).
- Establishing a network of maternal health referral centers (long-term goals).

The diagnostic phase serves as the foundation for effective transformation in healthcare settings. By thoroughly assessing the specific needs and challenges of the environment, organizations can create and execute strategic initiatives that result in significant and lasting improvements.

Key elements of this phase include leadership, strategic thinking, and powerful analytical tools, ensuring that transformation aligns with organizational objectives and meets the evolving demands of the healthcare landscape.

CULTURAL TRANSFORMATION AND EMPOWERMENT: INSIGHTS FROM RATAN JALAN

Transforming healthcare organizations requires fostering a culture that drives high energy, ownership, teamwork, and a commitment to continuous learning. According to Mr. Ratan Jalan, cultural transformation and empowerment are pivotal for sustainable healthcare transformation. The key elements include:

1. Defining the Desired Culture

- **High Energy and Ownership**: A dynamic environment where individuals are motivated to take initiative and responsibility is foundational.
- **Teamwork and Learning**: A collaborative spirit must coexist with a focus on personal and collective growth. Teams should collaborate to innovate and improve, fostering an environment of mutual respect and shared objectives.
- **Healthy Competition**: Encouraging constructive and balanced competition can drive performance while

emphasizing the importance of collective success over individual achievements.

2. Role Modeling: Leaders play a critical role in shaping and reinforcing the desired cultural norms by consistently embodying the organization's core values. They must:

- **Demonstrate Transparency:** Maintain open communication to build trust and clarity.
- **Ensure Fairness:** Apply policies and decisions equitably across all levels of the organization.
- **Hold Accountability:** Lead by example, take responsibility for outcomes, and encourage others to do the same.

3. Empowerment: Empowering employees is vital to fostering innovation and resilience in healthcare settings. This involves:

- **Delegating Authority:** Providing teams with the autonomy to make decisions within their areas of expertise.
- **Fostering Accountability:** Encouraging individuals to take ownership of their roles and outcomes.
- **Avoiding Centralization Pitfalls:** By decentralizing decision-making, organizations can enhance efficiency, creativity, and team confidence, reducing bottlenecks and over-reliance on leadership.

Transformation Through Collaboration and Support

1. Stakeholder Alignment: Mr. Jalan emphasizes the necessity of achieving internal alignment before seeking external collaboration. This involves:

- **Building Internal Trust:** Authenticity in communication and actions fosters trust among employees and leadership.
- **Precise Planning:** A well-articulated vision and roadmap are crucial for gaining stakeholders' buy-in.

2. Global and Political Support: For healthcare transformations to be impactful, they must align with both global frameworks and national priorities. Key considerations include:

- **International Guidance**: Leveraging frameworks and best practices from organizations like the WHO to inform strategies.
- **Political Incentives**: National and local government support can drive momentum by integrating healthcare transformations into broader public health agendas.

3. Sustainability of Change: Ensuring that transformation efforts are enduring requires a holistic approach:

- **Cultural Acceptance**: Long-term success is tied to embedding change within the organization's cultural fabric.
- **Leadership Consistency**: Sustained transformation is supported by leaders who consistently reinforce the vision and values of the change initiative.
- **Systemic Alignment**: Aligning processes, structures, and resources with the desired outcomes ensures that the transformation becomes self-sustaining over time.

Mr. Ratan Jalan's insights underscore the importance of cultural transformation, stakeholder alignment, and collaborative support in driving healthcare innovation. Empowering teams, aligning with global and political priorities, and embedding change into organizational culture are critical steps in achieving sustainable and impactful healthcare transformation.

MONITORING AND ADJUSTING TRANSFORMATION STRATEGIES

Effective transformation in healthcare requires continuous monitoring and evaluation (M&E) to ensure that change initiatives achieve their intended outcomes. Leadership and Change Management (LCM) processes incorporate robust mechanisms to track progress, identify barriers, and enable adjustments to strategies as needed.

This approach ensures alignment with organizational objectives and the evolving needs of healthcare systems.

Monitoring Transformation Strategies

Monitoring transformation strategies involves systematically tracking implementation progress, assessing performance against predefined metrics, and gathering feedback from stakeholders.

1. **Establishing Clear Metrics**
   - **Input Metrics**: Measure resources allocated to the change initiative (e.g., budget, staff training hours).
   - **Process Metrics**: Evaluate the efficiency and fidelity of implementation (e.g., adherence to new workflows, engagement levels).
   - **Outcome Metrics**: Focus on results such as improved patient care, reduced costs, or enhanced staff satisfaction.

2. **Utilizing Pilot Programs:** Piloting initiatives enables organizations to test changes on a smaller scale, identify potential challenges, and gather data to refine strategies before implementing them on a full scale. **For example**, implementing a new electronic health record (EHR) system in one department before rolling it out hospital-wide.

3. **Stakeholder Feedback:** Gathering insights from physicians, nurses, administrative staff, and patients ensures that the transformation aligns with their needs and concerns. Feedback mechanisms may include:
   - Surveys and interviews.
   - Feedback sessions during team meetings.

4. **Leveraging Technology:** Advanced tools, such as dashboards and analytics platforms, provide real-time data on transformation progress, allowing healthcare leaders to track key performance indicators (KPIs) effectively.

Adjusting Transformation Strategies

Adjustments are critical to addressing challenges and enhancing the effectiveness of change initiatives. Flexibility in LCM enables healthcare organizations to respond to unforeseen barriers and evolving needs.

1. Continuous Evaluation: Regular assessments using M&E frameworks help identify gaps and areas for improvement. The evaluation focuses on:

- Progress toward defined goals.
- Barriers to implementation.
- Unexpected outcomes or resistance.

2. Root Cause Analysis: When progress stalls, conducting a root cause analysis can help identify underlying issues, such as:

- Inadequate training.
- Communication gaps.
- Resource constraints.

3. Adaptive Leadership: Leaders play a pivotal role in driving adjustments. Key practices include:

- Maintaining open communication channels with teams.
- Empowering staff to propose solutions and improvements.
- Revisiting the vision and ensuring alignment with organizational objectives.

By integrating effective monitoring and adaptive strategies, healthcare organizations can ensure that transformation initiatives remain relevant, sustainable, and capable of delivering long-term improvements in patient care and operational efficiency.

4. Iterative Pilots and Scaling: Based on feedback and data, pilot programs can be iteratively adjusted before being implemented on a full scale. For instance, adjusting a telemedicine rollout strategy based on feedback from initial users.

5. Reassessing Metrics: As initiatives evolve, the original metrics may need refinement. New KPIs can be added to reflect changing priorities or unexpected results.

TOOLS AND FRAMEWORKS FOR MONITORING AND ADJUSTING

- **Change Management Metrics**
  - **Adoption Rates**: Measure the percentage of employees actively using new systems or processes.
  - **Compliance Rates**: Evaluate adherence to new workflows or protocols.
  - **Employee and Patient Satisfaction**: Conduct regular surveys to gauge stakeholder sentiment and engagement.
- **Dashboards and Data Visualization:** Tools like Tableau or custom healthcare analytics platforms enable real-time visualization of progress against KPIs, to have a deeper insight into Business Analytics and Intelligence units to monitor the trends, progress, and predictive analytics for various context requirements
- **Feedback Mechanisms:** Digital platforms such as Zendesk or AI-driven survey tools facilitate anonymous feedback and suggestions from staff and patients. Employee Feedback mechanisms, Community Feedback tools
- **Scientific Frameworks**
  - **Utilize frameworks** like **Theory of Change** (TOC), **Log Frame, Monitoring, Evaluation & Learning Tools** (MEL), **Prosci's ADKAR Model**, or any change model framework to monitor individual and organizational readiness for change.
  - Incorporate insights from research (e.g., ScienceDirect) to benchmark progress against industry standards.

Monitoring and adjusting transformation strategies are integral to the success of healthcare change initiatives. By leveraging robust monitoring and evaluation (M&E) frameworks, collecting feedback, and maintaining flexibility, healthcare organizations can ensure their strategies remain effective and aligned with evolving goals. The dynamic nature of healthcare demands continuous improvement, making adaptive change management a cornerstone of sustainable transformation.

NATIONAL-LEVEL HEALTHCARE TRANSFORMATION: INSIGHTS FROM Dr ALKA PARIKH

Effective healthcare transformation at a national level requires a focus on equitable access, affordability, and proactive public health measures. Dr. Alka Parikh emphasizes three core principles for achieving meaningful change:

1. Accessibility and Affordability: A cornerstone of successful national healthcare strategies is ensuring that services are both affordable and accessible to all segments of the population. This involves reducing financial barriers to care and addressing regional disparities in healthcare availability. Policies and programs must bridge gaps between urban and rural areas, ensuring that underserved communities can access essential services.

2. Prioritizing Sanitation and Prevention: Dr Alka advocates for public health systems that emphasize sanitation and preventive measures. By addressing sanitation infrastructure, nations can significantly reduce the burden of communicable diseases. Proactive measures, such as immunization campaigns and preparedness for disease outbreaks, create resilient systems that can effectively mitigate health crises.

3. Learning from Global Examples: Drawing inspiration from global success stories, Dr Alka highlights how countries with varying economic capacities have achieved remarkable healthcare outcomes through targeted investments:

- **China**: Strategic improvements in infrastructure and healthcare systems have enabled widespread access and improved health indicators.
- **Sri Lanka**, despite its relatively low GDP, demonstrates how limited resources can be effectively utilized to build a robust healthcare system, underscoring the importance of prioritization and efficiency.

These examples illustrate that economic wealth is not the sole determinant of healthcare success. Instead, deliberate planning, resource optimization, and sustained commitment can yield transformative results.

National-level healthcare transformation presents a multifaceted challenge that requires an integrated approach. By focusing on accessibility, sanitation, and prevention and leveraging lessons from global models, governments can substantially improve health outcomes for their populations.

TRANSFORMING HEALTHCARE SYSTEMS WITH LEADERSHIP AND CHANGE MANAGEMENT

Transforming healthcare systems to meet evolving demands requires the effective integration of leadership and change management (LCM) principles. Leadership provides the vision, direction, and motivation to initiate change, while change management ensures the structured implementation and sustainability of that change. Together, they are the cornerstone of successful transformation efforts in diverse healthcare settings.

Leadership as a Catalyst for Transformation: Effective healthcare leaders inspire change by setting clear goals, fostering a shared vision, and maintaining a focus on patient-centered care. They embody essential values such as transparency, accountability, and inclusivity, cultivating an environment where teams feel valued and empowered. Leadership extends beyond individuals at the top; it encompasses champions at every level who drive change by embodying and reinforcing the organization's goals and values.

Key Leadership Strategies for Healthcare Transformation

- **Visionary Thinking**: Anticipating future trends and aligning organizational goals with emerging healthcare needs.
- **Stakeholder Engagement**: Building trust and fostering collaboration across clinical, administrative, and policy domains.
- **Adaptability**: Responding to challenges with resilience and innovation, ensuring the organization remains agile in dynamic environments.

THE ROLE OF CHANGE MANAGEMENT

Change management offers a framework for converting visionary leadership into practical strategies. It addresses the specific challenges that arise from critical decision-making, diverse teams, and long-standing practices in healthcare. Effective change management involves organized processes that guide organizations through the planning, implementation, and assessment stages.

Core Components of Effective Change Management

- **Diagnostic Phase**: Assessing the healthcare setting's needs, challenges, and readiness for change.
- **Stakeholder Alignment**: Ensuring internal and external stakeholders understand and support transformation initiatives.
- **Piloting and Scaling**: Testing and refining strategies in controlled environments before full-scale implementation.

- **Monitoring and Evaluation (M&E)**: Tracking progress through measurable indicators and adjusting based on outcomes.

Bridging Leadership and Change Management: For healthcare transformation to succeed, leadership and change management must operate in tandem:

- **Cultural Transformation**: Leaders foster a culture of collaboration, accountability, and continuous improvement, while change management embeds these values into daily operations.
- **Empowering Teams**: Delegating decision-making authority to frontline teams ensures that changes are practical and effective at the operational level.
- **Overcoming Resistance**: Leaders address resistance by demonstrating the benefits of change, while change management systematically identifies and mitigates sources of opposition.

Sustainability of Transformation: Sustaining change in healthcare requires a long-term commitment to cultural, systemic, and structural alignment. Leaders must ensure that change initiatives are institutionalized through:

- **Continuous Learning**: Encouraging knowledge sharing, training, and adaptation to new practices.
- **Policy Integration**: Embedding changes into organizational policies, ensuring consistency and adherence.
- **Feedback Loops**: Utilizing real-time data and stakeholder feedback to refine processes and maintain momentum.

THE FUTURE OF LEADERSHIP AND CHANGE MANAGEMENT IN HEALTHCARE

As healthcare systems face increasing pressures from aging populations, technological advancements, and rising patient expectations, the role of leadership and change management will only grow in importance.

Integrating data-driven decision-making, patient-centric approaches, and global best practices will enhance their effectiveness.

Transforming healthcare is essential and challenging, requiring visionary leadership and effective change management. Together, these components build resilient, adaptable, and high-performing healthcare systems that deliver quality care in an ever-evolving landscape.

6

NAVIGATING CAREER GROWTH IN HEALTHCARE LEADERSHIP & CHANGE MANAGEMENT

Healthcare is a dynamic and ever-evolving field, driven by technological advancements, shifting patient demographics, regulatory changes, and the growing complexity of care delivery systems. This environment presents abundant career growth opportunities, particularly for those aspiring to transition into leadership roles. A career in healthcare leadership provides the opportunity to shape the future of healthcare systems, influence patient outcomes, and drive organizational success. However, the leadership journey is not without its challenges. It demands a multifaceted approach that goes beyond clinical expertise or technical knowledge, requiring strategic acumen, emotional intelligence, adaptability, and the ability to inspire and manage change.

THE HEALTHCARE LANDSCAPE: OPPORTUNITIES FOR GROWTH

Healthcare leadership is a broad domain that encompasses hospital administration, public health management, policy advocacy, and leadership roles within pharmaceutical companies and healthcare technology firms.

With an aging global population, the rising prevalence of chronic diseases, and rapid technological innovation, the demand for skilled leaders has never been higher.

Opportunities for Career Growth in Healthcare Leadership

- **Diverse Career Paths**: Healthcare leaders can specialize in operations, finance, patient care quality, or human resources within healthcare organizations.
- **Impactful Work**: Leadership roles empower professionals to make informed strategic decisions that enhance patient care and operational efficiency.
- **Global Opportunities**: The universal nature of healthcare creates international demand, offering diverse cross-cultural career prospects.

However, achieving leadership roles requires deliberate preparation. Leadership is not solely about authority—it is about influence, collaboration, and driving sustainable change.

ESSENTIAL SKILLS FOR HEALTHCARE LEADERSHIP

While clinical expertise forms the foundation for many healthcare professionals, it alone does not guarantee leadership success. Aspiring leaders must develop a diverse set of skills to navigate the complexities of organizational, financial, and technological challenges.

Key Competencies for Healthcare Leaders

- **Strategic Thinking**: Understanding how to align organizational goals with the broader vision of healthcare delivery.
- **Emotional Intelligence**: Developing self-awareness, empathy, and interpersonal skills to manage diverse teams and patient populations effectively.

- **Change Management**: Leading organizational transformation in response to new technologies, regulatory changes, or shifting patient needs.
- **Financial Acumen**: Understanding budgeting, cost control, and financial planning to ensure organizational sustainability.
- **Effective Communication**: Articulating visions, motivating teams, and engaging stakeholders at all levels.
- **Data-Driven Decision-Making**: Leveraging analytics to make informed decisions and measure outcomes.

In addition, healthcare leaders must be prepared to manage crises, foster innovation, and create inclusive environments that enable teams to thrive.

COMMON CHALLENGES IN HEALTHCARE LEADERSHIP

- **Rapid Technological Advancements**: Leaders must stay ahead of emerging technologies, such as AI, telemedicine, and electronic health records (EHRs), while ensuring that patient-centered care remains a priority.
- **Regulatory and Ethical Pressures**: Balancing compliance with legal and ethical standards while maintaining high-quality care is a continuous challenge.
- **Workforce Dynamics**: Managing a diverse, interdisciplinary workforce requires cultural sensitivity and collaborative strategies.
- **Burnout and Stress**: Healthcare professionals often face high-stress levels; leaders must prioritize the well-being of both themselves and their teams.

Recognizing and preparing for these challenges is crucial for anyone aspiring to lead in the healthcare sector.

Healthcare leadership is an exciting and impactful career path, offering endless opportunities for growth, innovation, and meaningful contributions to patient care and organizational success. By developing key leadership competencies, embracing change, and navigating challenges with resilience, aspiring leaders can drive transformation in one of the world's most critical industries.

BUILDING A LEADERSHIP FOUNDATION

Healthcare leadership often begins with small yet impactful steps, such as assuming supervisory roles, joining committees, or leading small-scale projects. These experiences provide a strong foundation for understanding team management, decision-making, and resource allocation.

Aspiring leaders should actively seek opportunities to demonstrate initiative, such as:

- Spearheading quality improvement initiatives within their organizations.
- Contributing to strategic planning efforts that enhance patient care and operational efficiency.

Navigating Change in Healthcare

Change is a constant in healthcare—whether it's implementing a new electronic health record (EHR) system, expanding telemedicine services, or responding to a public health crisis.

Leaders must:

- Guide their organizations through transitions while minimizing disruption. To do so, they must implement change management strategies, such as:
- Involving key stakeholders early in the process.
- Maintaining transparent communication to foster trust.
- Creating a culture of adaptability that embraces innovation.

UNDERSTANDING THE LEADERSHIP LANDSCAPE IN HEALTHCARE

Achieving leadership in healthcare is both challenging and rewarding. By developing critical skills, employing effective strategies, and committing to lifelong learning, healthcare professionals can lead confidently and drive meaningful change.

In the upcoming sections, we will explore the essential requirements for excelling in healthcare leadership, equipping you with the tools and insights to make a lasting impact on your organization and the broader healthcare community.

The Diversity of Healthcare Leadership Roles

The healthcare sector offers a variety of leadership roles, each contributing uniquely to the system's efficiency and success. These roles can be categorized into:

- Clinical Leadership
- Administrative Leadership
- Healthcare Program Policy and Strategic Leadership

1. **Clinical Leadership:** Clinical leaders bridge the gap between direct patient care and organizational goals. They work on the frontlines, ensuring high-quality care delivery while engaging in broader initiatives to improve processes and outcomes.

- **Common Clinical Leadership Roles**
  - **Medical Directors**: Oversee clinical departments, ensuring standards of care, regulatory compliance, and the integration of evidence-based practices.
  - **Nurse Leaders**: Manage nursing teams, advocate for patient safety, and drive quality improvement initiatives.
  - **Specialty Unit Leaders**: Supervise specific areas like intensive care, oncology, or pediatrics, ensuring that specialized care is delivered effectively.

Each of these roles requires a unique combination of clinical expertise, leadership skills, and a commitment to innovation and excellence.

2. **Administrative Leadership:** Administrative leaders focus on the operational, financial, and strategic aspects of healthcare organizations. Their roles are essential for maintaining efficiency and sustainability.

   - **Examples of Administrative Leadership Roles**
     - ○ **Hospital Administrators**: Oversee the day-to-day operations of hospitals, including budgeting, staffing, and regulatory compliance.
     - ○ **Healthcare Managers**: Manage specific services or departments, such as human resources, IT, or logistics, within healthcare organizations.
     - ○ **Chief Operating Officers (COOs):** Implement strategic plans and oversee the operational performance of healthcare systems.

3. **Healthcare Program, Policy, and Strategic Leadership:** Leaders in this domain work at a macro level to influence healthcare policy, public health initiatives, and system-wide improvements.

   - **Examples of Healthcare Program, Policy, and Strategic Leadership Roles**
     - ○ **Health Policy Makers**: Develop and advocate for regulations and policies to improve public health and access to care.
     - ○ **Public Health Leaders**: Address population health challenges through programs targeting disease prevention and health promotion.
     - ○ **Chief Executive Officers (CEOs)**: Lead entire healthcare organizations, setting strategic visions and ensuring alignment with long-term goals.

Each of these roles demands a unique combination of skills, experiences, and qualifications, making the healthcare leadership landscape both challenging and rewarding.

ESSENTIAL SKILLS FOR HEALTHCARE LEADERS

While the specific skills required may vary by role, successful healthcare leaders generally share core competencies that enable them to excel in their positions. These skills fall into three primary categories:

i. Technical Skills

- **Healthcare Knowledge** – A deep understanding of healthcare systems, clinical workflows, and patient needs.
- **Financial Acumen** – Proficiency in budgeting, financial planning, and resource allocation.
- **Data-Driven Decision Making** – The ability to interpret analytics and metrics to guide organizational strategies.
- **Regulatory Compliance** – Familiarity with healthcare laws, accreditation requirements, and ethical standards.

ii. Interpersonal Skills

- **Communication** – Effective leaders articulate their visions clearly and listen actively to feedback.
- **Emotional Intelligence** – Building trust and managing relationships with empathy and self-awareness.
- **Team Building** – Fostering collaboration among multidisciplinary teams and resolving conflicts constructively.
- **Change Management** – Guiding teams through transitions, such as adopting new technologies or shifting policies.

iii. Conceptual Skills

- **Strategic Thinking** – The ability to see the bigger picture and align departmental or organizational goals with broader objectives.
- **Problem-Solving** – Tackling complex challenges with innovative and evidence-based solutions.

- **Visionary Leadership** – Inspiring teams to pursue long-term goals while adapting to short-term needs.

Pathways to Leadership: Building Experience and Expertise

Becoming a healthcare leader requires a thoughtful and diverse approach to career advancement.

This path typically includes:

- Acquiring relevant experience
- Building leadership skills
- Seeking further education or certifications

1. Gaining Relevant Experience: Hands-on experience in clinical or administrative roles provides a strong foundation for leadership.

- **Clinical Leaders** – Many begin as physicians, nurses, or allied health professionals, gaining firsthand insight into patient care before transitioning into leadership.
- **Administrative Leaders** – Entry-level administrative positions or project management roles help professionals understand the operational aspects of healthcare organizations.
- **Public Health Leaders** – to start with, program research associate, policy and program implementation areas, at least to gain experience with various public health, government, policy institutions, NGO, and catalyst organisations

2. Developing Leadership Competencies: Leadership skills can be honed through a combination of:

- Practical experience
- Mentorship
- Formal training

Key steps include:

1. Leading Projects – Taking charge of quality improvement initiatives, research projects, or departmental changes.

2. Participating in Committees – Engaging in decision-making bodies to gain exposure to organizational strategy and policy development.

3. Seeking Mentorship – Learning from experienced leaders who can provide guidance, feedback, and networking opportunities.

4. Pursuing Education and Certifications: Advanced education is often necessary for healthcare leadership roles.

- **Master's Degree Program**s such as:
  - Master's in Healthcare Administration (MHA)
  - Master's in Business Administration (MBA) with a healthcare focus
  - Master's in Public Health (MPH)
  - Master's in Public Policy
  - Master's in Health Financing and Economics
  - Master's in Health Informatics
- **Short-term programs/certifications**: There are various short-term programs offered online, by governments, the WHO, and significant policy institutions; some of them are listed below
  - **Coursera Public Health Courses (Global)**: Offers free and paid courses (e.g., Epidemiology, Global Health Policy) from universities like UC Berkeley and Yale—over 100 courses, with certificates.
  - **The Global Health Network Training Centre (Global)**: Provides free eLearning (4.1 million modules taken by 785,000 users) on research skills, proposal writing, and disease prevention. Available in multiple languages, supporting preventive care
  - **WHO Open WHO (Global)**: Free courses on pandemics, malaria, and health emergencies. Trained 1Million workers, critical for crisis response
  - **ECDC Fellowship Programme (Europe)**: Includes EPIET (Intervention Epidemiology) and

EUPHEM (Public Health Microbiology) tracks. Trains specialists in outbreak response, supporting 150+ countries.

o **TEPHINET Field Epidemiology Training Programs (FETPs, Global)**: Operates in 150+ countries, training 12,000+ epidemiologists. Example: Uganda's FETP reduced Ebola cases by 90% in DRC (2018–2020).

o **Public Health Foundation (PHF, USA)**: Offers TRAIN Learning Network, with courses on performance management and immunization. Serves 6,000+ professionals in 79 countries.

o **National Institute of Public Health Training and Research (NIPHTR, India)**: Provides short-term courses for paramedics (e.g., ANMs, Community Health Guides) and an MPH program. Focuses on hospital management and preventive care.

These degrees provide professionals with specialized knowledge in healthcare management, finance, and policy development. The healthcare leadership field is diverse and challenging. From clinical directors to policymakers, each role allows influencing patient care and organizational success. Aspiring leaders should develop various skills, acquire relevant experience, and embrace lifelong learning to succeed in this dynamic environment.

Types of Healthcare Management Roles in Hospitals
i. Practice Management: Practice managers oversee the day-to-day operations of medical practices, including doctors' offices and specialty clinics. Their duties include:
- Overseeing administrative tasks like payroll and employee reviews.
- Developing strategies to improve service delivery.
- Addressing challenges that arise within the practice.

ii. Clinical Coordination: Clinical coordinators work closely with healthcare providers to maintain care standards and ensure patient satisfaction. Their responsibilities include:

- Developing and implementing patient care plans.
- Ensuring compliance with industry regulations during inspections and audits.
- Managing resource allocation for medical supplies and equipment.

iii. Finance Management: Financial managers focus on the monetary health of healthcare organizations. Their tasks include:

- Budget planning and oversight.
- Managing payroll and benefits systems.
- Preparing financial reports for stakeholders and regulatory bodies.

iv. Operations Management: Operations managers ensure that a healthcare organization's physical and administrative infrastructure runs smoothly. Key duties include:

- Supervising support staff and administrative teams.
- Managing medical records and regulatory compliance documentation.
- Leading operational projects, such as opening new units or implementing new technologies.

v. General Management: General managers oversee comprehensive operations within healthcare organizations. Depending on the size of the organization, its scope of work may involve:

- Strategic planning and corporate management.
- Handling both clinical and non-clinical aspects of service delivery.
- Managing relationships with external stakeholders, such as government agencies or industry partners.

vi. Project Management: In healthcare, project managers drive specific initiatives, such as developing new treatments or implementing public health campaigns. Their responsibilities often include:

- Allocating resources and coordinating team efforts.
- Establishing timelines and benchmarks for project milestones.
- Reporting progress to executives or governing bodies.

Types of Healthcare Management Roles in Public Health

a) **Health Policy Analyst/Advisor**
  - **Description**: Develop and evaluate policies to strengthen health systems and allocate resources.
  - **Responsibilities**: Advise governments, draft legislation, and assess policy impact (e.g., universal health coverage).
  - **Key Skills**: Policy analysis, stakeholder engagement, economics.

b) **Public Health Program Manager**
  - **Description**: Plan, implement, and evaluate programs (e.g., vaccination, nutrition) to achieve health goals.
  - **Responsibilities**: Manage budgets, coordinate teams, and monitor outcomes.
  - **Key Skills**: Project management, monitoring and evaluation, leadership.

c) **Health Communication Specialist**
  - **Description:** Design campaigns to promote health behaviors and counter misinformation.
  - **Responsibilities:** Create educational materials, engage media, and use digital platforms.
  - **Key Skills:** Messaging, behavioral science, digital marketing.

d) **Global Health Specialist**
  - **Description**: Coordinate international health initiatives, focusing on cross-border issues like pandemics.
  - **Responsibilities**: Collaborate with WHO, NGOs, and governments; secure funding.

- **Key Skills**: Diplomacy, grant writing, program design.

e) **Public Health Research Coordinator**
- **Description**: Manages research projects, coordinating teams, budgets, and timelines.
- **Responsibilities**:
- Oversee study implementation, from ethics approval to data collection.
- Liaise with stakeholders (e.g., WHO, local health ministries).
- Ensure research aligns with community needs.
- **Key Skills**: Project management, grant writing, stakeholder engagement.

f) **Health Data Analyst/Biostatistician**
- **Description**: Analyzes complex health datasets to identify trends and evaluate program impacts.
- **Responsibilities**:
- Apply statistical models (e.g., regression, survival analysis) to assess intervention outcomes.
- Create data visualizations for policymakers (e.g., dashboards).
- Ensure data quality and ethical compliance.
- **Key Skills**: Programming (Python, SAS), data visualization (Tableau), epidemiology.

STEPS TO ENTER HEALTHCARE MANAGEMENT

Healthcare management roles typically require a combination of academic qualifications, practical experience, and interpersonal skills. Below are the steps to enter this field:

1. Pursue Relevant Education: While a medical degree is not necessary, a background in healthcare administration or business management is often essential. Most common educational paths include a Bachelor's Degree in Healthcare Management or Business Administration, or Advanced degrees like a Master's in Healthcare Administration (MHA) or a healthcare-focused MBA or a healthcare focused policy management

2. Gain Practical Experience: Practical exposure is essential for understanding the unique challenges and workflows of the healthcare industry. Aspiring healthcare managers can gain experience through:

- Internships or volunteer work in hospitals, clinics, and healthcare programs
- Entry-level roles in healthcare organizations, such as an administrative assistant or a department coordinator position, and as a public health researcher or a program associate

3. Apply for Graduate Schemes or Internships: Many healthcare organizations offer graduate schemes targeting recent graduates. These programs provide:

- Structured training
- Mentorship
- Pathways to permanent employment

4. Create a Professional CV and Cover Letter: A compelling application should:

- Highlight relevant education, internships, and experiences that demonstrate leadership potential and a commitment to healthcare.
- Tailor each application to the specific role, emphasizing the skills and experiences most relevant to the job description.

5. Apply for Entry-Level Management Roles: Start by applying for positions like:

- Department Manager
- Operations Assistant
- Project Coordinator
- Public Health Manager

These roles offer opportunities to:
- Learn the intricacies of healthcare management
- Build a professional network
- Gain hands-on leadership experience

HEALTHCARE MANAGER DUTIES

1. Overseeing Operations: At Hospital or Public Health program locations.
- Coordinate clinical and nonclinical activities, such as scheduling, administrative workflows, and quality assurance checks, to ensure seamless operations.
- In a similar way for program location, a public health manager would look for administrative review across village-level health units, primary health centers, and hospitals; the program being managed will also have a bearing on the role and duties

2. Financial Oversight: Manage budgets, monitor expenditures, and prepare financial reports to maintain the financial health of healthcare organizations.

3. Human Resource Management: Oversee recruitment, training, and performance evaluation to build and maintain effective teams.

4. Developing and Implementing Initiatives: Lead projects to improve care delivery, increase operational efficiency, or address community health needs.

5. Ensuring Compliance and Quality: Conduct risk assessments and respond to audits to ensure that healthcare organizations meet industry standards and comply with relevant legal requirements.

6. Liaising with Stakeholders: Interact with investors, government agencies, and industry boards to align organizational goals with external expectations.

EFFECTIVE STRATEGIES FOR ADVANCING HEALTHCARE LEADERSHIP

Advancing in healthcare leadership requires a combination of practical experience, formal education, and strategic relationship-building. The healthcare industry is complex and constantly changing, and leaders must possess a unique blend of technical skills, emotional intelligence, and strategic thinking. While the path to leadership in healthcare may vary depending on individual aspirations and organizational structures, several strategies have been identified as particularly effective in helping healthcare professionals advance into leadership roles. These strategies are rooted in on-the-job experiences, formal education, and mentorship, all of which contribute to developing the multifaceted skill set required for success in healthcare leadership.

On-the-Job Projects and Leading Teams

One of the most effective ways to advance healthcare leadership is through hands-on experience. Healthcare professionals who assume leadership roles within projects, particularly those involving team leadership, acquire critical skills and knowledge that cannot be replicated in a classroom setting. Leading teams provides exposure to real-world challenges, enabling leaders to develop problem-solving abilities, improve communication, and gain insights into the practical applications of theoretical concepts.

- **Leading Cross-Functional Teams:** One of the most significant opportunities for growth is leading cross-functional teams. In healthcare, these teams often consist of individuals from diverse departments, including medical staff, administrative teams, and finance professionals. Leading such a team requires a strategic mindset, the ability to manage diverse perspectives, and the skill to drive collaboration across different disciplines.

By managing these teams, healthcare leaders develop the skills to navigate complex organizational dynamics, resolve conflicts, and deliver results that benefit the entire organization.

- **Project Management**: Healthcare leaders who manage projects—whether related to process improvement, new technology integration, or patient care initiatives—develop critical leadership capabilities. These projects provide opportunities to hone time-management skills, budget allocation, and resource management, all of which are key to effective healthcare leadership. Furthermore, project management enables leaders to recognize the importance of delivering results on time, managing stakeholder expectations, and ensuring that every aspect of the project aligns with the organization's mission and strategic objectives.

Exposure to Different Positions within the Organization

Another highly effective strategy for advancing healthcare leadership is gaining exposure to different organizational positions. Many healthcare leaders find that moving through various roles in different departments helps them gain a comprehensive understanding of how healthcare organizations function.

- **Rotational Programs**: Some healthcare organizations offer rotational programs that allow individuals to work in various departments or healthcare settings for a specified period. These programs provide future leaders with a 360-degree view of the organization, enabling them to understand the unique challenges and opportunities in each area. Whether working in clinical operations, finance, human resources, or strategic planning, exposure to different positions fosters a deeper understanding of organizational needs and enhances decision-making skills.

- **Observing Senior Leaders**: Shadowing senior leaders within the organization is an effective strategy. By observing experienced leaders, aspiring healthcare professionals gain valuable insights into navigating complex situations, managing pressure, and making informed, critical decisions. This process enables individuals to absorb various leadership styles, communication techniques, and management strategies vital for their professional development.

Formal Training and Education

While hands-on experience is invaluable, formal education remains essential to advancing healthcare leadership. Formal training programs—ranging from short-term courses to medium-term certifications—are designed to equip healthcare professionals with the skills and knowledge necessary to address the industry's evolving challenges.

- **Short-Term and Medium-Term Courses**: Many healthcare organizations offer short-term courses and workshops that focus on leadership skills, management techniques, and specific areas such as finance, operations, or healthcare technology. Experts often lead these courses in the field and can offer healthcare professionals practical tools and frameworks that can be directly applied to their leadership roles. Medium-term courses, such as certifications or diplomas in healthcare management, offer a deeper exploration of the theoretical aspects of healthcare leadership, enabling individuals to develop the strategic and operational thinking necessary for senior leadership roles.

- **Advanced Degrees**: Pursuing advanced degrees, such as a Master of Healthcare Administration (MHA) or an MBA with a healthcare focus, is another effective strategy for advancing healthcare leadership. These degrees provide a comprehensive understanding of the healthcare system, business principles, and leadership strategies. The formal structure of such programs enables professionals to establish a solid foundation in subjects such as finance, organizational analysis, strategic planning, and human resource management—all of which are essential for effective leadership in the healthcare field.

Coaching and Mentoring

Coaching and mentoring are two of the most effective strategies for developing healthcare leadership. By partnering with a coach or mentor, emerging leaders gain personalized insights, receive constructive feedback, and build long-term relationships with senior leaders who can offer guidance and support.

- **Executive Coaching**: Executive coaching is often tailored to healthcare professionals in leadership roles or those aspiring to move into leadership positions. A coach helps individuals refine their leadership style, develop communication skills, and navigate organizational challenges. Executive coaching can also provide a safe space for leaders to explore their strengths and weaknesses, allowing for growth in emotional intelligence, conflict resolution, and strategic decision-making.
- **Mentorship Programs**: Mentorship programs enable emerging leaders to establish relationships with experienced leaders who can provide guidance, advice, and career support. Mentors offer valuable

insights into how to approach leadership challenges, and they can help mentees establish a professional network. Mentoring relationships often evolve, fostering a sense of trust and mutual respect that benefits both parties. Mentors help mentees develop both the technical aspects of leadership and the softer skills essential in healthcare, such as empathy, resilience, and emotional intelligence.

Practical Scenarios and Problem-Solving Exercises

Engaging in real-world situations and problem-solving tasks is crucial for healthcare leaders. In the intricate healthcare sector, characterized by high stakes and rapid pace, leaders must effectively possess critical thinking and practical problem-solving skills.

- **Case Studies**: Case studies offer aspiring healthcare leaders the chance to analyse real-life situations and apply their knowledge to practical scenarios. By discussing case studies, leaders can explore various approaches to problem-solving, examine the consequences of different decisions, and gain insight into how other leaders have addressed similar challenges. Case studies provide a platform for collaborative learning, enabling leaders to engage in discussions that offer diverse viewpoints and insights.
- **Simulation Exercises**: Healthcare leaders gain from simulation exercises that replicate real-life crises or organizational challenges. These activities enable leaders to practice decision-making, teamwork, and crisis management in a safe environment, helping them enhance their skills without the stress of actual consequences. Simulation exercises serve as valuable training tools for leadership teams, boosting their capability to

handle emergencies and unforeseen situations in healthcare settings.

Data-Driven Decision Making

Data-driven decision-making is essential for modern healthcare leadership. With vast healthcare data, leaders are better equipped to make informed decisions that improve patient care, operational efficiency, and financial outcomes. Using data to guide decisions allows leaders to measure progress, identify areas for improvement, and adjust strategies accordingly.

- **Capacity Building and Team Development**: Healthcare leaders who 291nalyse data to uncover performance gaps and training requirements can take focused action to enhance their teams' capabilities. Leaders can introduce training programs that address challenges and enhance team performance by leveraging insights into staff performance, patient outcomes, and operational efficiency.

- **Strategic Planning and Stakeholder Management**: Leaders who use data in their strategic planning processes can make more informed decisions that align with organizational goals and address stakeholder concerns. Data-driven decision-making enables healthcare leaders to anticipate trends, optimize resource allocation, and foster stakeholder engagement, ensuring the organization achieves both short-term and long-term objectives.

COACHING AND MENTORSHIP IN HEALTHCARE LEADERSHIP

Coaching and mentorship play pivotal roles in the career progression of healthcare professionals who aspire to leadership positions.

Both processes provide emerging leaders with invaluable insights, guidance, and support in a highly demanding and unpredictable environment.

Why Coaching and Mentorship Matter?

a) **Knowledge Transfer and Professional Development**: One primary benefit of coaching and mentorship is knowledge transfer. Senior leaders often have a wealth of experience, from navigating organizational politics to managing crises and making high-stakes decisions. Emerging leaders can learn from these experiences, gaining valuable insights into handling challenges that may not be covered in formal education. Mentorship enables leaders to refine their skills, such as strategic thinking, emotional intelligence, and decision-making.

b) **Personalized Guidance and Reflection**: Unlike traditional training programs, coaching and mentorship offer personalized, one-on-one guidance tailored to the individual's needs and challenges. Coaches and mentors are often able to offer feedback that helps individuals reflect on their leadership style, strengths, and areas for improvement. This tailored guidance helps mentees develop self-awareness, a crucial skill for effective leadership.

c) **Building a Strong Network**: Mentors and coaches typically bring a network of professional contacts. By connecting their mentees with others in the field, they facilitate valuable networking opportunities that might otherwise be difficult to access. These connections can open doors for career advancement, partnerships, or collaborative efforts that benefit professional and organizational growth.

CONTINUOUS LEARNING AND ADAPTATION IN HEALTHCARE LEADERSHIP

Healthcare leaders face ever-evolving challenges driven by external factors (such as regulatory changes, technological advancements, and demographic shifts) and internal factors (such as changes in organizational structure, employee expectations, and patient needs). To sustain a leadership career and continue delivering results, healthcare leaders must prioritize continuous learning and adaptation.

Why Continuous Learning is Crucial?
a) **Adapting to Industry Changes**: Healthcare is one of the most rapidly changing industries. New technologies, treatment protocols, regulatory standards, and funding models frequently emerge, meaning healthcare leaders must proactively update their knowledge and skills. Without continuous learning, healthcare leaders risk falling behind in managing these changes and maintaining organizational effectiveness.
b) **Staying Competitive in a Dynamic Field**: Healthcare leaders must demonstrate high competency and innovation to remain competitive. Continuous learning through formal education, certifications, and self-directed study ensures that leaders remain competitive within the field. Furthermore, it helps them to meet the increasing demands for efficiency, patient satisfaction, and cost-

effectiveness—critical expectations in today's healthcare environment.

c) **Developing New Skills:** As healthcare organizations evolve, their leaders must also evolve. Continuous learning enables leaders to acquire new skills essential for addressing emerging challenges, such as understanding the complexities of healthcare data analytics, leading virtual teams, or implementing patient-centric care models. Healthcare leaders who keep pace with developments in these areas are more likely to advance in their careers.

Example 1: Embracing Telemedicine: The COVID-19 pandemic dramatically accelerated the adoption of telemedicine in healthcare settings. Healthcare leaders who could adapt quickly to this change, by implementing telemedicine platforms, ensuring patient confidentiality, and training staff, were better positioned to manage patient care during the pandemic. For example, Maria, the CEO of a regional hospital, had already adopted telemedicine as a strategic initiative even before the pandemic struck. Her proactive approach to integrating new technologies into her healthcare organization allowed her to ensure continuity of care during the crisis, resulting in increased patient satisfaction and the continuation of critical services.

Example 2: Data-Driven Decision Making: Given the increasing reliance on healthcare data for decision-making, healthcare leaders must adapt by becoming proficient in data analytics. For example, David, the Chief Financial Officer (CFO) of an extensive hospital system, successfully led the transition to data-driven budgeting. By continuously learning about financial forecasting tools and data analysis techniques, David was able to optimize resource allocation, reduce costs, and improve the hospital's financial outcomes.

TYPICAL CAREER PATHS LEADING TO HEALTHCARE LEADERSHIP

Healthcare leadership careers typically follow structured and dynamic paths. As professionals accumulate experience and expertise, they advance through different roles. This progression usually depends on education, mentorship, hands-on experience, and networking.

Common Career Trajectories in Healthcare Leadership

Clinical Leadership Pathway
Step 1: Clinical Expertise - Many healthcare leaders begin their careers in clinical positions, such as doctors, nurses, or therapists. This clinical expertise serves as the cornerstone of their leadership paths.

Step 2: Managerial Roles - After gaining experience in clinical practice, numerous individuals transition to managerial positions, such as clinical coordinators or department heads.

Step 3: Executive Roles - With continued leadership development, some clinicians transition into senior roles, such as Chief Medical Officer (CMO) or Chief Nursing Officer (CNO). In these roles, they oversee the clinical operations of healthcare organizations, shaping policies and ensuring the delivery of high-quality patient care.

Administrative Leadership Pathway
Step 1: Entry-Level Healthcare Administration – Individuals entering healthcare administration often begin their careers as office managers, healthcare administrators, or department heads.

Step 2: Mid-Level Management – As they accumulate experience, healthcare professionals in administration often advance to roles such as Director of Operations or Vice President of Administration.

Step 3: Senior Leadership – With further career development, some move into high-level executive roles such as Chief Executive Officer (CEO), Chief Operating Officer (COO), or Chief Financial Officer (CFO), where they are responsible for the overall strategic direction and management of healthcare organizations.

Public Health Leadership Pathways
A) Policy and Advocacy Pathway

- **Focus**: Develop, implement, and advocate for health policies to strengthen systems and address inequities.
- **Entry-Level Roles**:
  - **Policy Analyst Intern**: Researches health policies for NGOs or ministries. Example: Supporting Rwanda's vaccination policy (UNICEF, 2021).
  - **Health Communication Assistant**: Creates campaign materials. Example: Nigeria's polio radio campaigns (WHO Africa Report, 2022).
- **Mid-Level Roles**:
  - **Health Policy Analyst/Advisor**: Drafts legislation and evaluates impacts. Example: Ethiopia's advisors shaped HEP, reducing maternal mortality by 50% (WHO, 2020)
  - **Health Equity Advocate**: Promotes inclusive policies. Example: Kenya's advocates raised female health managers by 10% (Global Health Action, 2023)
- **Senior-Level Roles**:
  - **Policy Director/Chief Advisor**: Leads national or global health strategies. Example: Dr. Agnes Binagwaho's policies achieved 93% immunization coverage (The Lancet Global Health, 2020).

B) Leadership and Administration Pathway

- **Focus**: Guide health organizations, systems, or policies through strategic leadership and resource mobilization.
- **Entry-Level Roles**:
  - **Health Administrator**: Manages clinic operations or budgets. Example: Haiti's PIH administrators supported TB care (PIH Report, 2022).
  - **Program Coordinator**: Assists with large-scale projects. Example: Rwanda's vaccination coordinators (UNICEF, 2021).
- **Mid-Level Roles**:
  - **Health Systems Manager**: Oversees facilities or programs. Example: Ethiopia's HEP managers reduced malaria by 40% (WHO, 2020).
  - **Global Health Specialist**: Coordinates international initiatives. Example: Moeti's Ebola response in Africa (Bulletin of WHO, 2019).
- **Senior-Level Roles**:
  - **Executive Director/Chief Health Officer**: Leads organizations or ministries. Example: Dr. Tedros led Ethiopia's health reforms, scaling up the number of Community Health Workers (CHWs) to 40,000 (*The Lancet Global Health*, 2020).

C) Public Health Researcher Pathway

- **Entry-Level Roles**
  - **Research Assistant**: Supports study design, data collection, and literature reviews. Example: Assisting malaria surveillance in Ethiopia, contributing to a 40% incidence reduction (*WHO, 2020*).
  - **Field Epidemiologist Trainee (FETP)**: Conducts basic outbreak investigations under

supervision. Example: Nigeria's FETP trainees tracked cholera, reducing cases by 25% (*TEPHINET Report*, 2020).

- **Data Analyst Intern**: Performs preliminary data cleaning and analysis. Example: Supporting Rwanda's vaccination data analysis (*UNICEF, 2021*).

- **Mid-Level Roles**
  - **Research Epidemiologist**: Designs and leads studies (e.g., cohort, case-control). Example: Rwanda's epidemiologists studied HPV vaccination, achieving 90% uptake (UNICEF, 2021).
  - **Health Data Analyst/Biostatistician**: Conducts advanced statistical analyses. Example: Butaro Hospital analysts improved cancer treatment adherence by 30% (The Lancet Oncology, 2021).
  - **Implementation Scientist**: Evaluates program scalability. Example: India's ASHA program evaluation raised maternal care by 20% (Health Systems & Reform, 2022).
  - **Social and Behavioral Scientist**: Researches health behaviors. Example: Haiti's PIH scientists reduced TB stigma, resulting in a 50% reduction in mortality (BMJ Global Health, 2019).
  - **Health Equity Researcher**: Analyzes disparities. Example: Kenya's researchers boosted female health access by 10% (Global Health Action, 2023).

- **Senior-Level Roles**
  - **Principal Investigator/Global Health Researcher**: Leads multicountry studies and shapes global policies. Example: Dr. Matshidiso

Moeti's polio research raised Africa's vaccination coverage to 80% (WHO Africa Report, 2022).

- ○ **Research Program Director**: Oversees research portfolios for organizations or ministries. Example: Rwanda's Butaro Hospital director scaled cancer research, achieving 90% chemotherapy adherence (*The Lancet Oncology*, 2021).
- ○ **Chief Scientific Officer**: Guides national or international research agendas. Example: Dr. Agnes Binagwaho's research leadership informed Rwanda's 93% immunization coverage (*The Lancet Global Health*, 2020).

Academic or Research-Based Leadership: Professionals in this pathway may begin their careers in academic positions or as researchers, gaining expertise in healthcare policies, systems, or clinical practices. Over time, they may move into leadership positions in academic institutions, healthcare think tanks, or government agencies, influencing healthcare policy and innovation.

NETWORKING IN HEALTHCARE CAREER ADVANCEMENT

Networking plays a crucial role in career advancement across all fields, but it holds particular significance in healthcare due to its collaborative and interconnected nature. It goes beyond merely accumulating contacts; it focuses on fostering authentic, mutually advantageous relationships that can unlock career opportunities, facilitate mentorship, and deliver valuable perspectives on emerging challenges and trends.

The Importance of Networking in Healthcare

1. Access to Career Opportunities: Networking enables healthcare professionals to discover career opportunities that may not be publicly advertised. Many leadership positions in healthcare organizations are filled through internal promotions or word-of-mouth referrals. A solid professional network increases the likelihood of being considered for these opportunities. Leaders and decision-makers in healthcare organizations tend to hire individuals they know or have interacted with in professional settings.

2. Mentorship and Guidance: Networking provides access to mentorship from individuals who have successfully navigated similar career paths. By connecting with experienced professionals, emerging leaders can gain advice, feedback, and support, which can significantly accelerate their career trajectory. Mentors can help guide healthcare professionals through complex organizational politics, leadership challenges, and decision-making processes.

3. Collaboration and Knowledge Exchange: Healthcare professionals, particularly those in leadership positions, must stay updated with industry developments, new technologies, and emerging best practices. Networking with colleagues, peers, and experts allows professionals to exchange knowledge and stay informed. It also provides opportunities for collaboration on projects, research, and initiatives that can enhance one's professional reputation and career growth.

4. Building a Reputation: Networking helps healthcare professionals build a reputation within their field. Individuals can become recognized as thought leaders by attending conferences, speaking at industry events, and engaging with peers in professional organizations. This visibility can lead to career advancements, such as invitations to serve on boards, advisory committees, or as a consultant for other healthcare institutions.

5. Support During Career Transitions: Career transitions, whether moving from a clinical to an administrative role or shifting to a leadership position, can be challenging. A strong network can provide guidance and reassurance during these transitions. Networking with others who have undergone similar shifts can offer valuable insights into navigating challenges, such as adjusting to new roles or developing new skill sets.

Strategies for Effective Networking in Healthcare

1. Engage in Professional Associations: Joining professional organizations can significantly expand a healthcare leader's network, offering access to industry insights, collaborations, mentorship, and thought leadership platforms. These associations often host conferences, webinars, and workshops, and provide avenues to publish, speak, and contribute to strategic dialogues.

2. International and Regional Associations

- International Hospital Federation (IHF)
- Asia Pacific Healthcare Forum (APHF)
- Middle East Healthcare Leadership Congress
- Council for Health Service Accreditation of Southern Africa (COHSASA)
- National Accreditation Board for Hospitals and Healthcare Providers (NABH)
- Association of Healthcare Providers – India (AHPI)
- Healthcare Federation of India (NATHEALTH)
- American College of Healthcare Executives (ACHE)
- Healthcare Financial Management Association (HFMA)
- American Medical Group Association (AMGA)
- National Association for Healthcare Quality (NAHQ)

3. Institute for Healthcare Improvement (IHI) – Innovation in healthcare quality and patient safety. Attend Industry Events and Conferences: Attending or speaking at healthcare-related conferences, summits, and webinars is an excellent way to connect with other professionals and industry leaders. Networking at these events can help individuals stay up-to-date with industry trends, meet potential mentors, and discover new career opportunities.

4. Build and Maintain Relationships: Networking is not just about attending events; it's about nurturing relationships over time. Maintaining contact with colleagues, former professors, and mentors through occasional emails, social media interactions, or meetings can help keep connections strong. Building lasting relationships increases the chances of receiving career recommendations or being invited to new opportunities.

5. Leverage Social Media and Professional Platforms: Platforms like LinkedIn have become integral tools for professional networking and career advancement. Healthcare professionals can use LinkedIn to showcase their skills, connect with peers, share industry insights, and engage in professional discussions. Active participation in relevant LinkedIn groups or online forums can further extend networking opportunities.

BALANCING CLINICAL RESPONSIBILITIES WITH LEADERSHIP AMBITIONS

Healthcare professionals seeking leadership roles face a significant challenge in balancing their clinical duties with the demands of leadership development. Those in clinical positions, such as physicians, nurses, or therapists, are often heavily focused on patient care, which hinders their ability to cultivate the leadership skills essential for advancing their careers.

- **Seek Out Leadership Opportunities within Clinical Roles**: One way to balance clinical responsibilities with leadership ambitions is to seek out leadership opportunities within the clinical environment. For example, a physician could take on a role as a clinical director, department head, or lead physician, which provides exposure to leadership responsibilities while still being involved in patient care. Nurses can also pursue leadership roles, such as nurse manager or clinical coordinator, which enable them to integrate clinical practice with leadership functions.

- **Pursue Incremental Leadership Training**: Healthcare professionals can develop their leadership skills through incremental steps, starting with shorter leadership courses or certifications. These can be tailored to fit around clinical responsibilities. For example, attending evening or online courses in healthcare management, leadership skills, or team dynamics can help build knowledge without interfering with clinical hours.

- **Utilize Mentorship and Coaching**: Mentorship and coaching can help balance clinical and leadership duties. Mentors can offer guidance on how to balance time and prioritize tasks effectively. They can help healthcare professionals understand how to assume leadership responsibilities gradually while maintaining high standards in patient care. Regular coaching sessions can ensure professionals stay on track toward their leadership ambitions without sacrificing their clinical commitments.

- **Delegate Clinical Tasks When Possible**: Healthcare professionals should assign specific clinical responsibilities to their teammates to create room for leadership duties. For example, nurses and doctors can guide junior staff or train peers, allowing them to share their clinical responsibilities while embracing leadership roles within the team. This delegation helps balance clinical and leadership responsibilities, encouraging a collaborative atmosphere where team members feel empowered to take on leadership roles.

- **Time Management and Prioritization**: Healthcare professionals aspiring to leadership must be adept at managing their time and prioritizing tasks.

Strategies such as scheduling specific times for leadership development activities, setting clear goals, and delegating tasks help create the space needed for professional growth. Utilizing tools like time-blocking for educational activities or leadership meetings can ensure clinical duties do not interfere with leadership goals.

- **Explore Healthcare Leadership Programs**: Numerous healthcare systems provide leadership development initiatives that enable clinicians to enhance their leadership capabilities while continuing their clinical duties. These programs typically offer organized training, mentorship opportunities, and insights into administrative tasks, helping professionals acquire leadership experience while remaining in their clinical positions.

CASE STUDY: EXPLORING CLINICAL LEADERSHIP IN THE UK HEALTHCARE SECTOR

Clinical leadership has gained increasing recognition in healthcare systems worldwide, particularly in the United Kingdom (UK), where clinicians are being encouraged to take on leadership roles. Given the complex demands of healthcare, the involvement of healthcare professionals, particularly doctors, in leadership roles is seen as essential for driving change and improving patient outcomes. However, while there is significant literature on clinical leadership, little research has focused on understanding how senior healthcare leaders perceive the term and the essential qualities for success. This case study explores the findings from a qualitative study conducted by Nicol, Mohanna, and Cowpe (2011), which aimed to capture the views of senior healthcare leaders in the UK about the evolving concept of clinical leadership and the necessary attributes for effective leadership within the NHS (National Health Service).

Study Overview

The study was conducted between 2010 and 2011, involving 20 senior healthcare leaders from various sectors of the UK healthcare system. Participants included NHS executives, chief executives from strategic health authorities, medical directors, former health ministers, medical deans, and key figures in the field of medical leadership. The research aimed to understand how these senior leaders define clinical leadership, the changing attitudes toward leadership roles, and the attributes necessary for success in the ever-evolving healthcare environment.

The study utilized semi-structured interviews and grounded theory methodology to identify key themes from the interviews. This qualitative approach enabled an in-depth exploration of the perceptions, challenges, and future directions of clinical leadership within the UK healthcare system.

Key Findings: The study uncovered several significant findings related to clinical leadership, its evolving role in the NHS, and the qualities required for success in leadership positions. The following sections outline the key themes that emerged from the research.

1. Changing Attitudes Towards Clinical Leadership

One of the most striking findings from the study was the evidence of shifting attitudes toward clinical leadership, particularly among doctors and healthcare trainees. Historically, doctors in the UK, especially junior doctors, were not typically inclined to take on leadership roles. There was a prevailing view that medical professionals should focus on clinical practice and leave the management and leadership tasks to administrators. However, the study revealed that attitudes were changing, with increasing numbers of young doctors expressing interest in taking on leadership roles within healthcare organizations.

This change can be attributed to several factors, including a growing recognition that clinical leaders can influence patient care, shape organizational culture, and contribute to the efficiency of healthcare systems. Senior healthcare leaders reported that trainees and junior doctors were increasingly encouraged to engage in leadership development activities, such as participating in management training programs, assuming leadership roles within their departments, and becoming involved in decision-making processes. This shift aligns with the broader trend of encouraging healthcare professionals to take on leadership roles, ensuring the NHS remains responsive to the needs of patients and the public.

2. Ambiguity Surrounding the Term 'Clinical Leadership'

Despite the growing interest in clinical leadership, there was considerable unease among the study participants about the ambiguity of the term 'clinical leadership.' Many senior healthcare leaders felt that the definition of clinical leadership was unclear and that it often seemed to be a doctor-centric term. They highlighted that the role of a clinical leader is not well understood, and its boundaries are difficult to define. This ambiguity can lead to confusion about what clinical leadership entails and who should be responsible for it.

Several leaders argued that the term 'healthcare leadership' might be more inclusive and better reflect the collaborative nature of leadership in healthcare settings. Healthcare leadership, they suggested, should encompass a broader range of professionals, including doctors, nurses, allied health professionals, and administrators, all of whom contribute to the effective functioning of healthcare organizations. The idea of healthcare leadership being more inclusive aligns with the concept of fostering a multidisciplinary approach to healthcare management, where all team members, regardless of their professional background, share responsibility for leading and improving patient care.

3. Attributes and Skills Required for Success in Healthcare Leadership

Despite the uncertainty around the precise definition of

clinical leadership, there was broad agreement among senior healthcare leaders regarding the key attributes and skills required for effective leadership in healthcare settings. The study participants identified several core competencies that are essential for success in leadership roles: Communication Skills: Effective communication was consistently cited as one of the most critical attributes for healthcare leaders. The ability to communicate, listen actively, and engage with colleagues at all levels of the organization is vital for fostering collaboration, building trust, and ensuring that organizational goals are aligned with patient needs. Decision-Making: Healthcare leaders are often required to make difficult decisions under pressure. Making informed, timely decisions is essential for ensuring that patient care is not compromised and that the organization functions efficiently.

Emotional Intelligence: Healthcare leaders must possess high emotional intelligence (EI) to navigate complex interpersonal dynamics and manage conflicts effectively. EI enables leaders to understand and regulate their own emotions and those of others, which is particularly important in high-stress healthcare environments. Vision and Strategic Thinking: Healthcare leaders must be able to think strategically and have a clear vision for the future of their organizations. This involves anticipating challenges, identifying opportunities for improvement, and leading change initiatives that enhance patient care and organizational performance.

Adaptability: Given the rapidly changing healthcare environment, leaders must be adaptable and open to innovation. The ability to adopt new technologies, policies, and practices is crucial for delivering high-quality care and enhancing healthcare delivery.

Team Building and Collaboration: Effective healthcare leadership requires building and managing teams. Leaders must be able to inspire, motivate, and empower their teams, fostering a culture of collaboration and mutual respect.

4. The Role of Historical and Political Context in Leadership

Another significant finding from the study was the importance of understanding the historical and political context in which healthcare leadership is situated. Senior healthcare leaders emphasized that successful leadership in the NHS requires an awareness of the political and organizational structures that shape healthcare delivery. The evolving nature of healthcare policy, funding mechanisms, and organizational priorities presents challenges for leaders, making it essential to navigate these factors effectively.

Leaders must be attuned to the political landscape, as decisions made by government bodies and regulatory agencies have a direct impact on healthcare organizations. Moreover, understanding the historical context of the NHS—its values, culture, and mission—can help leaders stay grounded in the principles that guide the organization and ensure that changes are made in ways that align with its core values.

5. The Need for Investment in Leadership Development

The study concluded that, while the attributes required for effective healthcare leadership are well understood, significant investment in leadership development is necessary to harness the leadership potential within the NHS fully. Participants argued that a dedicated Healthcare Academy or similar institution could provide the necessary infrastructure for training and developing future healthcare leaders. This would enable leaders at all levels to enhance their skills, engage in leadership research, and contribute to a broader conversation about the future of healthcare leadership.

The study by Nicol, Mohanna, and Cowpe (2011) provides valuable insights into the evolving nature of clinical leadership in the UK healthcare sector. While there is growing interest among clinicians in taking on leadership roles, there is still uncertainty surrounding the term 'clinical leadership' and its implications.

Senior healthcare leaders agree on the essential attributes and skills required for success in leadership, including communication, decision-making, emotional intelligence, and adaptability. Furthermore, they emphasize the importance of understanding the historical and political context in which leadership operates and call for increased investment in leadership development to ensure that the NHS can effectively meet future challenges.

This case study underscores the necessity for a more inclusive and comprehensive approach to leadership in healthcare, one that acknowledges the contributions of all professionals and promotes a collaborative, multidisciplinary environment. By investing in leadership development and embracing a broader definition of leadership, healthcare organizations can better position themselves to improve patient care and navigate the complexities of the modern healthcare landscape.

Reference: Nicol, E. D., Mohanna, K., & Cowpe, J. (2011). Perspectives on clinical leadership: A qualitative study exploring the views of senior healthcare leaders in the UK. Clinical Leadership Academy, Clinical Education Centre, Staffordshire ST4 6QG, UK.

A ROADMAP FOR ASPIRING HEALTHCARE LEADERS

Embarking on a career in healthcare leadership is both a challenging and rewarding endeavor. The healthcare industry is dynamic, multifaceted, and continually evolving, offering numerous opportunities for those passionate about enhancing patient outcomes and shaping the future of healthcare delivery. As someone at the beginning of your journey toward healthcare leadership, it is essential to understand not only the broad scope of leadership in healthcare but also the personal and professional qualities required to succeed.

1. Develop a Strong Foundation in Healthcare Knowledge and Skills

The first step in any leadership journey is building a solid foundation of knowledge and expertise. Healthcare leadership requires a deep understanding of clinical practices, healthcare systems, organizational structures, policies, and regulations. While leadership abilities are critical, effective leaders must also grasp the complexities of the healthcare industry.

To begin, focus on acquiring relevant educational qualifications. Most healthcare leadership roles require a background in healthcare management, public health, or a related field of study. A Bachelor's degree in healthcare administration, nursing, or medicine can be an essential starting point. For those aiming to pursue senior leadership positions, obtaining advanced degrees such as a Master of Healthcare Administration (MHA), a Master of Business Administration (MBA) with a healthcare focus, or a Master of Public Health (MPH) is highly recommended. These qualifications will equip you with the technical knowledge and skills necessary to manage healthcare organizations and make informed decisions effectively.

Equally important is developing core competencies related to healthcare systems, such as finance, quality improvement, patient safety, policy analysis, and ethics. These competencies will provide the critical foundation upon which you can build your leadership abilities. You can obtain this expertise through formal education, certifications, and continuous learning.

2. Gain Practical Experience Through Diverse Roles

Healthcare leadership is not just about theory and academic qualifications but also about gaining practical experience and understanding the realities of healthcare delivery. As a budding leader, you must seek opportunities to work in various aspects of healthcare. Whether through clinical, administrative, or management roles, gaining exposure to different healthcare settings will allow you to learn the intricacies of the system, build a broad skill set, and prepare you for leadership responsibilities.

One of the most effective ways to gain experience is to take on roles that challenge you. For instance, starting as a healthcare manager, team leader, or assistant in a clinical or administrative setting can provide you with firsthand insight into how healthcare organizations operate. Working in diverse settings, such as hospitals, primary care, long-term care, and public health organizations, will help you understand the various components of healthcare delivery. Take the opportunity to learn from experienced colleagues and mentors who can guide you in managing projects, overseeing operations, or leading teams.

As you progress, seek roles with increasing responsibility, such as department head or director of a specific function.

These roles will expose you to leadership challenges, including budgeting, policy-making, and organizational development. The ability to handle complex projects, manage multidisciplinary teams, and solve problems in real-world scenarios will be critical as you work toward higher leadership positions.

3. Develop Emotional Intelligence and People Management Skills

One of the most essential attributes of a successful healthcare leader is emotional intelligence (EI). Healthcare leadership is inherently people-centered, and leaders must be able to manage relationships, foster collaboration, and resolve conflicts effectively. Emotional intelligence enables leaders to recognize and manage their own emotions as well as those of others, thereby facilitating effective communication and informed decision-making.

Leaders with high emotional intelligence (EI) are better equipped to navigate the complex interpersonal dynamics of healthcare teams. They can motivate, inspire, and guide staff while maintaining a positive and supportive work environment.

To develop emotional intelligence, practice self-awareness, empathy, and active listening. Additionally, build resilience to manage stress and maintain composure in high-pressure situations, as healthcare environments can often be demanding and unpredictable.People management skills are also vital for any healthcare leader. As a leader, you must build, manage, and sustain high-performing teams. To excel, focus on fostering a culture of collaboration and mutual respect within your team. Invest time in developing your team members by providing them with the necessary resources, training, and opportunities for growth and development. Encourage open communication, and be proactive in addressing any challenges or concerns that arise within your team.

4. Build a Network of Mentors and Peers

No one achieves success in healthcare leadership alone. Building a network of mentors and peers is crucial for personal and professional growth. Mentorship is invaluable as it allows you to gain insights from individuals who have already walked your path. Mentors can provide advice, share their experiences, help you navigate challenging situations, and offer guidance as you make important career decisions.

When seeking mentors, look for experienced leaders who can provide both career-specific and leadership-focused guidance. It is also beneficial to find mentors who offer diverse perspectives, including clinical, operational, financial, and strategic. Additionally, actively engage with peers in the healthcare leadership space. Peer networks provide opportunities for collaboration, sharing best practices, and gaining different perspectives on common challenges.

Consider joining professional associations and leadership programs that offer opportunities for networking, continued education, and leadership development. Participating in events and forums dedicated to healthcare leadership can also provide exposure to new ideas, trends, and innovations.

5. Focus on Strategic Thinking and Change Management

Healthcare is constantly evolving, influenced by shifting policies, technological advancements, patient expectations, and financial pressures. Effective healthcare leaders must be strategic thinkers who can anticipate challenges, seize opportunities, and guide their organizations through change.

Begin by learning to think strategically about healthcare delivery. This means understanding both the long-term and short-term goals of your organization and aligning your actions with its mission and vision. Develop the skills to assess risks, make data-driven decisions, and lead organizational change initiatives. Healthcare leaders frequently must manage significant transitions, including the implementation of new technologies, changes in regulatory requirements, or shifts in patient care models. Your ability to lead during times of change will be tested as you face challenges that require innovative solutions and the support of your teams.

Mastering change management is key to successful leadership in healthcare. Change is inevitable, and your ability to lead teams through transitions while maintaining morale and ensuring continuity of care will set you apart as an effective leader.

Stay informed about emerging trends in healthcare, such as value-based care, digital health, and patient-centered models, and position yourself as someone who can drive these innovations.

6. Commit to Lifelong Learning and Adaptation

Healthcare leadership is not a static pursuit. As the industry continues to evolve, so must your skills and knowledge. As an aspiring healthcare leader, commit to lifelong learning and ongoing professional development. Stay current with the latest developments in healthcare policies, leadership practices, technology, and innovations. Participate in continuing education programs, leadership workshops, and conferences to refine your skills and expand your knowledge base.

Additionally, embrace the value of feedback. Actively seek feedback from colleagues, mentors, and team members to gain a better understanding of your strengths and areas for improvement. Reflect on your leadership style and make adjustments as necessary to better serve your team and organization.Healthcare systems are becoming increasingly complex, and as a leader, you must be adaptable to meet the demands of a dynamic environment. Your ability to learn, grow, and evolve will ensure that you are well-equipped to handle new challenges and maintain your effectiveness as a leader.

7. Lead with Integrity and a Focus on Patient-Centered Care

Finally, always lead with integrity. Healthcare leadership is grounded in the principle of improving patient outcomes, and this must remain your guiding focus. Strive to create a healthcare environment that prioritizes patient-centered care, where every decision you make is focused on enhancing the quality of care and the patient experience.

Healthcare leadership is not about personal recognition but about making a lasting impact on the lives of patients and the healthcare community. Maintain a strong sense of ethics, responsibility, and accountability as you guide your teams. A leader who values transparency, honesty, and collaboration will inspire confidence and loyalty in their teams and stakeholders.

As you embark on your journey toward healthcare leadership, remember that it is a path of continuous growth, learning, and adaptation. Equip yourself with the proper knowledge, gain hands-on experience, develop key leadership attributes, and build relationships with mentors and peers. With a strategic mindset, a commitment to lifelong learning, and a deep sense of purpose, you will be well on your way to becoming an impactful leader in healthcare, shaping the future of the industry and making a meaningful difference in the lives of patients and communities.

CONCLUSION

As we reach the end of this journey together, it's clear that the healthcare ecosystem is complex, ever-evolving, and, at times, daunting. However, it's equally evident that leadership and change management drive successful transformation.

Throughout this book, we've explored the multifaceted nature of healthcare and the importance of understanding its foundational principles to lead meaningful change. We've also examined the vital role of leadership and the specific tools and frameworks that can guide us through the transformation process. So, what's next?

- Understanding the healthcare ecosystem is essential for viewing challenges and opportunities. The landscape is a dynamic web of stakeholders, policies, patient needs, and technologies. Navigating this ecosystem is key to effective transformation and guidance through changes.

- We explored healthcare leadership, emphasizing that it's about inspiring and engaging teams, rather than just exercising authority. Leaders who foster trust and communicate well will drive sustainable transformation.

- However, leadership is not enough; change is difficult, and obstacles arise. Tools and frameworks for transformation are invaluable. Chapter 3 introduced models that help leaders implement change initiatives, serving as blueprints for success. With a strong foundation in change management, you can lead enduring change.

- Sustainability is the real challenge, as mentioned in Chapter 4. One-off changes won't last; transformation must be woven into the fabric of your organization. Sustainable change management ensures changes become embedded in your institution's DNA, fostering an environment where change is embraced.

- Transformation is a journey requiring continuous growth. Chapter 5 outlined how to apply leadership and change management principles in the healthcare setting. You now have actionable steps to tackle organizational shifts, policy overhauls, and cultural transformations, equipping you to tailor your approach.
- Finally, in Chapter 6, we discussed navigating career growth in healthcare leadership. This evolving field requires continual skill honing. Embrace learning, seek mentorship, and take leadership roles. The healthcare sector needs leaders at all levels who understand the importance, as your growth in leadership now will impact the organizations and communities you serve tomorrow.

What does this mean? Healthcare is undergoing rapid change, and effective leadership and change management are more crucial than ever. As you step into your role—whether as a professional, leader, or change agent—the skills from this book will empower you to drive necessary transformations in healthcare organizations. You're equipped to inspire change, lead purposefully, and create lasting impacts on those you serve.

Remember, you are the change leader. You have the power to shape the future of healthcare. Please embark on your journey by utilizing these tools and insights. Each small action you take will play a significant role in the broader goal of transforming healthcare. The difference you can make is immense, and it begins with you.

Thank you for allowing me to be part of your journey. The road ahead may be challenging, but with strong leadership and a commitment to sustainable change, you can help create a better, more adaptive, and more impactful healthcare system for the future.

Let's make it happen.

ABOUT THE AUTHOR

Girish Bommakanti is a distinguished healthcare leader with over two decades of expertise in health system strengthening, spanning both public and private sectors. He has a remarkable track record of transforming healthcare organizations and driving innovative solutions across South Asia, Southeast Asia, the Middle East, and North Africa (MENA). His professional journey reflects his unwavering commitment to enhancing healthcare delivery, advancing public health, and promoting leadership and change management.

Currently serving as the **Global Director of Operations and Growth** for ACCESS Health International, Girish oversees transformative health system programs. His leadership has been pivotal in integrating primary care, developing digital health solutions, healthcare delivery, health financing innovations, capacity building platform and strengthening non-communicable disease (NCD) management systems. Under his strategic direction, ACCESS Health has expanded its footprint and impact in regions critical to global health progress.

Previously, as Group CEO of Healthcare Services Limited, Girish led the transformation of hospitals and healthcare systems. He focused on improving operational efficiency, driving quality improvements, and implementing health financing solutions to achieve sustainable impact. He has also held senior leadership roles in renowned organizations like Apollo Hospitals, Gleneagles Global Hospitals, Manipal Hospitals and CARE Hospitals, where he successfully managed operations, profitability, and growth.

Alongside his role in hospital leadership, Girish has significantly advanced public health through innovative rural health models that have impacted over a million individuals in three Indian states.

These initiatives integrated community-based primary care with microinsurance solutions, showcasing his skill in tackling health disparities using scalable and sustainable methods.

Girish's academic credentials are as impressive as his professional achievements. He holds an Executive Program in Strategic Management from the **Indian Institute of Management, Kozhikode**, an Executive Certificate in Leadership and Change Management from **IIM Tiruchirappalli,** Master's in Healthcare Management from the **Tata Institute of Social Sciences** and a Masters in Business Administration **from Osmania University**. His educational foundation, combined with hands-on experience, has equipped him to address the multifaceted challenges of the healthcare sector.

Beyond his professional roles, Girish is a passionate mentor and trainer dedicated to building the next generation of healthcare leaders. He co-founded **Pro Health Skills,** which focuses on healthcare management trainings, and **Suigeneris Spanish Training Center**, which reflects his entrepreneurial spirit and commitment to lifelong learning. Girish's work has extended globally, with impactful initiatives in Nigeria, Egypt, Poland, the Caribbean, and Fiji during his tenure at Apollo Hospitals. His diverse experiences have shaped a comprehensive understanding of healthcare ecosystems, making him a trusted advisor on health policy, capacity building, and market access programs for lifesaving innovations.

With a career spanning continents and an unrelenting drive to improve healthcare systems, Girish Bommakanti is a beacon of leadership, innovation, and transformational change in the global health landscape."

www.ingramcontent.com/pod-product-compliance
Lightning Source LLC
Chambersburg PA
CBHW030638270326
41929CB00007B/123